Age is Just a Number

Age is Just a Number

What a 97-Year-Old Record-Breaker Can Teach Us About Growing Older

CHARLES EUGSTER

with Matt Whyman

sphere

SPHERE

First published in Great Britain in 2017 by Sphere

5 7 9 10 8 6

A CIP catalogue record for this book
is available from the British Library.

ISBN 978-0-7515-6537-9

Typeset in Bembo by M Rules
Printed and bound in Great Britain by
Clays Ltd, St Ives plc

Papers used by Little, Brown are from well-managed forests
and other responsible sources.

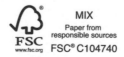

MIX
Paper from
responsible sources
FSC® C104740

Sphere
An imprint of
Little, Brown Book Group
Carmelite House
50 Victoria Embankment
London EC4Y 0DZ

An Hachette UK Company
www.hachette.co.uk

www.littlebrown.co.uk

Disclaimer

If you have any medical conditions or are not used to taking exercise, before undertaking any of the exercises in this book or changing your exercise regime, please discuss this with your GP or other medical practitioner. The information in the book is not intended to replace or conflict with the advice given to you by your GP or other health professionals. The author and publisher disclaim any liability directly or indirectly from the use of the material in this book by any person.

Prologue

Out of the Blocks

In the final moments before a sprint event, there's no such thing as silence. As I wait in my lane, considering the starting blocks and the two hundred metres oval I'm facing here, every cough and whisper is amplified. The same can be said for my heartbeat. Just then, as the race official draws breath to begin the start procedure, it feels to me like everyone can hear it thumping rapidly inside my chest.

'*On your marks . . .* '

The adrenalin rush is intense. It leaves me feeling like a stranger in my own body as much as in this environment. For this is my first visit to an indoor athletics track. Not only that, just to add to the pressure I'm racing in the

British Masters Championship. I make no bones about the fact that I'm a complete amateur. While my fellow competitors wear sleek, lightweight spikes, I've shown up in a pair of old trail shoes. I know nothing beyond self-taught technique. What I bring with me, however, is determination, enthusiasm and the will to win.

'Get set . . .'

At the start line, I simply plant one foot after the other and hope it looks like I know what I'm doing. Then I brace myself for the gun. By now, despite the cavernous space and the spectators filling the stands, I'm in a world of my own. The banked turns are my main concern. Earlier, I had one chance to walk the track. While the artificial surface felt quite alien to me, what surprised me most was the steepness of each curve. I simply have no idea of the technique required to enter and exit at full tilt. All I can do is hope it doesn't trip me up in every sense. Drawing each breath like it might be my last, I recognise that I'm in the hands of fate now.

The brutal crack of the starter's gun changes everything. In my mind, as I rise into the race, I'm transformed from a lamb into a lion and then a gazelle. With my legs and arms pumping, I'm up and running with as much power as I can muster. I gather momentum and velocity, and just hope my glasses stay in place.

It's not enough to stop the two runners in the outside lanes from effortlessly cruising ahead of me, but I'm not racing them. They're in a different age category. Even so, the fact that we're the only three on track speaks volumes.

From the age of fifty upwards, you would expect the field to dwindle. Remarkably, the two guys stretching away are in the 85–89 group. As for me, the sole entrant in the 95-plus club at ninety-six, I am literally in a class of my own.

The banked curve comes at me in a desperate blur. I keep my chin up, but thirty metres deep into this race my legs are beginning to complain. My mind receives the message and immediately translates it into failure. *I've come out too fast*, I think to myself. *I've blown it before I've barely begun.* As I clear the bank successfully and level on to the back straight, I should feel only relief. Instead, all of a sudden the track feels like it might go on for ever. Already the younger guys are approaching the second bank. I can't help but feel left behind and lonely. My heart is hammering so hard it feels like it might give out on me. I have a sudden urge to slow to a walk, a downshift in ambition as much as speed. I've come a long way to be here, in more ways than one, but with every breath it just feels like too little and far too late.

And then I pick up on something beyond the focus of my attention. It's taken me this far to realise that with the starter's pistol the crowd also came alive, but now I detect a name in the resonant cacophony of cheers, whoops and clapping, and that name belongs to me.

'Run, Eugster! You can do it! Go, Charles, go!'

If my legs have had enough by now, I realise I have to find what it takes in my spirit. It's all I have left. My style might have taken a turn for the worse, and I know for a fact that I'm not a gazelle but an old man close to his centenary year, but as the din from the spectators continues to build I feel their goodwill begin to carry me.

I will cross the finish line in the best time possible, I tell myself, even if it's the last thing that I do . . .

Now, there's a good chance that you consider the standout feature of this athletic venture to be my advanced age. Personally, I find it absurd that the video footage of my race you can find online has been viewed nearly one million times for the simple reason that I am old and healthy. In my view, it shouldn't be this way. I am not unique. I have simply made the most of what I have left, and I intend to share everything I've learned along the way so that you might follow in my footsteps – and even overtake me!

This is not a book devoted to running, I should say. That's just one of several recent passions that enable me to celebrate life. We often lose sight of this in our later decades, which is frankly both a shame and a waste. So in a sense this book is about *you* and *your* future. Even if it feels as if the sun is on the downswing, I'm here to demonstrate how it's possible to look forward to nothing but dazzling opportunities ahead.

Of course, in our modern world there is the less-than-attractive end game that we've been primed to expect, and that may well become a reality if you allow it to. I'm talking about an old age defined by frailty. Typically, such a day might begin with your carer opening the curtains and talking to you in loud, breezy but simplistic terms. They help you to sit up, oversee a trip to the bathroom, dress and then feed you before settling you in the sunny spot in the common room. Nobody talks very much. By and large your fellow care-home residents seem to inhabit their own memories. Still, you can always look forward to lunch. As long as it's mashed to a pulp you shouldn't have any difficulties. There's also visiting time in the afternoon. If you're lucky, a relative might pop in to see you, but they have busy lives to lead so they won't stay long. After that, you can expect a light supper and then bed, before this daily routine repeats until those curtains close for good.

I'm sure you'll agree, this isn't exactly a wonderful life scenario, and yet we've been conditioned to head towards this broken, dispiriting outcome as if we have no option.

I am here as living proof that it doesn't have to be this way. In fact, I'd like to show you how to make the rest of your life the best years you've ever had.

What you're about to read is designed to inspire as much as entertain, and ultimately encourage you to make a change for the better. If you're prepared to embrace the challenge then I can promise you great personal rewards. By taking one step at a time, and reviewing key aspects of your existence, you might start to see physical improvements at a stage when you thought everything could only go south. Perhaps more importantly, you'll find you're on the path to feeling good about yourself as you learn to live every day to the fullest.

Today, in my late nineties, I consider anyone in their sixties upwards to be teenagers in the world of old age. As we all know from experience, adolescence is about testing boundaries and working out what makes us tick. In my view, as we approach the autumn of our years we go through that phase all over again. The only difference is that we have the maturity, confidence and wisdom to make informed decisions. From experience, I can tell you that the potential to transform yourself for the better is mind-blowing. I can sum it up by asking three simple questions:

- Do you think that it's possible to be old without having any diseases or disability whatsoever, or even a cold?

- Is it too late to retrain or re-educate yourself, at a time when others are retiring, and go on to find gainful employment or even run a successful business?

- Can you imagine being fit enough at over ninety to be successful in international sporting competitions or even boast a beach-ready body?

Are these just dreams of the future?

No, the future is now, and I am living proof. I'm in fine health, and both hungry and able to take on new challenges. I take no medication, actively pursue all opportunities in work as well as sport, and feel more engaged with the world around me than ever before. I haven't always been in such good shape, however. This isn't about having unique genes or a lifelong commitment to a purist existence. In fact, there have been episodes in my life that could have led me to an early grave. In short, I'm just an old boy who refused to shuffle into decrepitude. At a time when I might have faced what I consider to be the horror of old age, I chose to reinvent myself. Now I'm here to light up that path for you.

I should say that along the way I've made plenty of mistakes. I've also been determined to pick myself up each time and learn lessons, which is the surest way that any of us grow wiser and more complete. In many ways I'm proud to account for those moments when I tripped over. It's all part of my journey, and helped to deliver me here so I might share my story as well as my strategies for making the most of later life. So, this is where we begin, as I revel in the wonder, the joy – and, yes – the *glory* of very old age.

Part One

First Life

1

A Weedy Boy Prone
to Headaches

My mother overfed me as a child. In doing so, I believe she saved my life. From a very early age, before I could walk and talk, I suffered a string of debilitating illnesses. From scarlet fever to whooping cough, mumps, chicken pox, measles, tonsillitis and German measles, it felt like I had them all. If it hadn't been for those excess fat reserves, insulating me at times of great weakness, I'm quite sure that I wouldn't have survived. In comparison to how I am today, I barely recognise that febrile little boy. I no longer even suffer a common cold, and yet in the beginning that kind of thing nearly finished me off.

I was born in London in the summer of 1919. The country was just emerging from the shadow of the First World War. If I do the sums, it's likely that I was conceived during the jubilant days that marked the armistice of the previous year. My father, Carl, who in his youth was a prominent football player, came from a Swiss family who had made their fortune in textiles. It was my grandmother who had urged him to settle in the English capital. She had been dispatched there herself as a younger lady in 1875. Taking residence in fashionable Holland Park, she spent a year attending dances and balls in the embrace of high society.

Carl arrived in the wake of a foray into cocoa production in West Africa, which collapsed due to outbreak of the First World War. Barely into his forties, and financially solvent, he decided on a change of pace to mark his new life in England. Accompanied by a strikingly beautiful Swiss lady of Polish descent named Josepha Antonia, who would become his wife and my mother, he took what we know today as 'early retirement'. This allowed him to pursue a passion for betting on the horses, though he never did so recklessly. He paid forensic attention to form and course, placing only small amounts of money on each-way bets and always covering his costs. Ironically for a gambler, he liked to minimise risk. I admired his sense of control.

'If I bet just a little bit more,' he would say, often drawing reflectively on a cigarette, 'then it won't work.'

My mother and father led a seemingly idyllic life, but it was one that had been marked by tragedy. Some years before my arrival, their first-born son succumbed to cot death. Inevitably, it influenced the way my parents regarded me when I came into the world. I was shown great love, but treated with some protectiveness and indulgence – not least when it came to food!

In between meals, and in the care of a nanny, I was pushed out in one of those high prams that were so popular at the time. Mine sported a yellow silk awning with fringes. We would go to Kensington Gardens, a popular haunt for nannies dressed in lovely uniforms with starched wide belts and long ribbons flowing from their caps. Their presence would often draw the attention of the guardsmen from the Palace. Impressive in their red uniforms and swagger sticks, and always working in pairs, they would flirt outrageously with these young women. Under the curious eyes of the infants in their care, the young ladies would laugh and chatter, while the guardsmen made the most of their time away from the parade ground. I remember those days with great fondness. I might not have learned to talk at the time, but it encouraged me to appreciate a pretty lady.

Throughout those early years my mother knitted all my clothes. She was a wonderful seamstress, and very creative. As well as my sailor's outfit, she dressed me in knee-high leather gaiters fastened with a long row of ball-shaped buttons. She even gave me a pageboy hair-style. I have always thought such attention formed the basis for my vanity. In later life, my focus on appearance would become a positive force by underpinning my commitment to staying in the best shape possible. At the time, however, I hated what she'd done with my hair. I felt it made me look like a girl.

We lived in a large flat with four rooms. It had hot and cold running water in the bathroom, which was considered a luxury, and two coal fires, as well as lino-leum floor covering and a gas stove (which looked like a strange insect on four legs). I was as well housed as I was well fed, and considered my parents to be quite wonderful. It was the constant bouts of illness that took the shine off my upbringing. When I think about why my immune system might have been so fragile, I do wonder whether my father's Herculean smoking habit was a contributory factor to my poor health. I suspect it might well have been linked to the premature death of my older brother, as well as a miscarriage my mother went on to suffer when I was still young before they stopped trying for another child. With some effort, my father could wait until after lunch before his first cigarette. After that, he would light the next one with the stub of the last and continue in this way throughout the rest of the day as if he was dependent on the smokes for oxygen. He bought his cigarettes in bulk, lived with nicotine-stained fingers and existed in a pungent fug. We had no idea that it could be such a harmful habit; not just in terms of the damage to his health but, through secondary smoke, to that of his loved ones. He would never have dreamed of hurting anyone. My father was the kindest person I have ever known, equal only to my mother, and I loved them both immensely.

Slowly, through those early years, I began to suffer less from illness and infection. I can only think my string of health battles had given me some immunity. Even so, I was left with a tendency to suffer intense and prolonged migraines. At times, it made my life a misery. If I could go just for half a day without a headache it would seem like heaven to me. I am also quite sure the experience stunted my growth. I went from being a podgy baby to a weedy boy prone to headaches. My best friend, who had always been much smaller than me, suddenly shot up and left me behind. I was desperate to feel better and be like everyone else.

That's when I began to wonder whether it would help if I took up a sport.

Aware of my desire to be more active, my parents entrusted my early education to the Froebel Educational Institute. This was a peculiar little school in West London that encouraged children to be individuals, as set out in the teaching principles established by its founder, the German pedagogue and inventor of the *Kindergarten*, Friedrich Froebel. When they first suggested this to me, six months before my schooling became compulsory at five, I kicked up such a fuss that the idea was quickly abandoned. As an only child, I had quickly learned the impact I could have by putting my foot down. It also proved my undoing when I finally attended the school, for I discovered that I had some catching up to do with classmates who had been there for half a year and could perform apparent miracles like look at a wall clock and tell the time correctly. Naturally, I blamed my parents for allowing me to overrule them in the first place.

As well as physical activity, the school encouraged music. This was something my mother and father dearly wished me to pursue. Unfortunately, a boy I befriended rather put me off by saying that music lessons were 'hell on earth'. Taking him at his word, I did my level best to avoid picking up an instrument, and this has always been a source of regret. Why? Because I believe music can have a profoundly beneficial effect on the brain throughout our lives. I am even inclined to believe the theory that it can enhance mathematical abilities as well as emotional wellbeing, but at the time even that wouldn't have persuaded me. I was just a little boy with bad migraines who hoped that being active would help him to escape such a curse. Music, at that moment and to my great regret, did nothing for me.

One of the guiding principles of the institute was the connection between hand, mind and heart. At a time when education was taught by rote, and enforced by corporal punishment, this created an unusually happy, engaging and creative environment for children. As well as traditional subjects such as language and science, we had lessons in everything from pottery to maypole dancing, play acting, gardening, weaving, knitting, cricket, football, Morris dancing and gymnastics, which was overseen by an instructress who always wore a black pleated skirt and would not begin without a cup of warm water to stir her. It might sound shocking now, when talking about primary education, but we were also encouraged to lace up boxing gloves. It was considered 'the noble art of self-defence' at the time, and if a little boy knew how to defend himself under the gentleman's rules of engagement then he would go far. Those gloves were so heavy it exhausted me just trying to swing a punch, but I enjoyed the physicality. Even if I didn't feel much better, and no doubt it made my headaches worse at times, it was a chance for me to unleash my frustration at feeling held back by my health.

Towards the end of my time at the school, we were encouraged to dress up as knights and ladies for a day of fun and games with a historical theme. To finish, we were permitted to pair off for a dance. As well as being feeble, I was cripplingly shy around the opposite sex. It meant I missed out on the opportunity to approach anyone attractive. I just waited until the braver boys had made their moves, which left me facing a dour Irish girl who reminded me of porridge made with water and served with salt. No doubt she took a similarly dim view of me, but as a knight to her lady we managed to endure the event in each other's company without saying much to one another. I never saw her again after we had left the school, but I'm always quick to tell the story of my early brief encounter with the great novelist Iris Murdoch, whose work I much admire.

Overall, I enjoyed being a pupil at this unconventional school. It broadened my horizons in many ways, but despite the emphasis on physical activity my headaches continued to bedevil me. They were such a constant distraction that my reports always stated that I could do better. I freely admit that during that time I perfected the art of doing only what was required in order to scrape an acceptable level of achievement. I'm sure I could have made more of an effort, but the migraines didn't help. It reached a point where I wondered if I might spend my entire life in misery. The experience ground me down, and perhaps paved the way for a deterioration in my health on reaching adolescence.

On one occasion, however, it proved to be my saving grace.

At thirteen, feeling rotten again, I was diagnosed with a case of severe tonsillitis. It was deemed that I should have my tonsils removed at a charity-run hospital. The nurses there were God-fearing, unpaid volunteers whose primary qualification was the Christian devotion of their humble lives to helping the sick. Their duties went so far as administering anaesthetic to the patients and assuring them everything would be fine. I had no issue when they put me under. What I do have is a vague memory of struggling on the table as the surgeon went in; sedated but not quite out for the count.

Despite such a traumatic experience, the procedure led to a profound change in my life that took us all by surprise. With my tonsils gone, my headaches simply stopped. After a childhood menaced by migraines, this torture I felt that I had suffered completely vanished. Not only did I feel much better, my body seemed to transform itself rapidly, as if finally permitted to catch up with my peers. I never quite reached the average size and height for my age, and yet the surging physical change I underwent came as a revelation. Brimming with energy and a confidence that I had never previously experienced, I developed a tendency to become quite boisterous. Perhaps it was my background in boxing, but I was even quick to pick a fight.

Through my young eyes, free from the tyranny of illness and infection at last, I had become *dynamite*.

2

On Water

In a bid to protect their only child, my parents would often address difficult, private or challenging subjects in my company by speaking in Swiss German. Driven by curiosity, and without letting on, I learned to pick up the language over time until I could understand every word they said. At times I had to keep a straight face listening to their intimate conversations, and I learned more about them than they ever imagined.

My mother's miscarriage, for example, followed a dark incident during a stay with her relations overseas. It involved an argument with her sister, so I learned, and a tumble down the stairs. I was never wise to whether she was pushed or fell, but it gravely affected her health. Prescribed morphine for pain relief, my mother quickly became dependent on her medication and effectively retreated from her former self. My father did his level best to take care of her, but life never regained the carefree air of my early years. At the same time, while life dimmed at home I found opportunities opening up for me elsewhere.

St Paul's School was only down the road in Hammersmith, but a world away from my Froebel education. It was bigger in every sense, teeming with older boys, and ruled by the cane. Having overcome a childhood marked by illness, I was keen to make my presence known. I set about this by spoiling for fights, an approach which came to an abrupt end when an older boy held my head and threatened to smash my face against a brick wall. Then there were my antics in the classroom, which is where I learned another vital lesson.

During the years 1934 to 1938, which spanned my time at St Paul's, I received the cane three times. I believe that qualifies me to speak as an expert on the subject of corporal punishment. I was never taken to task unjustly. In all three cases, in fact, I had behaved so abominably that I believe I thoroughly deserved what was coming to me.

On the first and second occasions the procedure

followed the usual ritual. Having caused a severe disruption in class, I was asked to stay behind after the lesson was over. Solemnly, my master told me to fetch the cane from the porter's lodge, where it was kept like some kind of religious artefact. I walked down the stairs to the lodge, which was situated on the right-hand side of the main entrance. At my request the porter gave me the cane and was gracious enough to wish me good luck.

I returned up the stairs with my heart beginning to kick. By this time, all the other members of the class had realised what was about to happen and had gathered outside the classroom door. Other boys who wished to enjoy the spectacle joined them. I made my way through the crowd, into the classroom where the master was waiting. He told me to close the door.

Outside, boys jostled for a peek through the keyhole. Others glued their ears to the door. Inside my punisher asked for the cane, told me to bend over a desk and instructed me to hold the hem of my jacket around my waist so that it wouldn't interfere with the procedure.

Masters at St Paul's were selected not only for their ability as teachers and sports coaches but also for their skill in using a cane. A good beater was one who was able to place the strokes parallel across the buttocks and as close to each other as possible. There was a teacher, whom I was fortunate enough not to come across, who went by the name of 'Chalky'. He would draw a line on the miscreant's bottom in chalk so that he would have a better chance of placing the strokes close together. This was considered by all of us to be grossly unfair. I would go so far as to say that it was cheating.

Without further word, the master commenced by giving me two strokes as hard as his strength would permit. The maximum number of permitted strokes was six. No one during my period at school, as far as I knew, ever received that amount – although one or two boys received four. Obviously, I didn't wish to give the master the pleasure of a cry or even a gasp of pain. I endured it in absolute silence. With the punishment over, he asked me to stand straight and then gave me the cane to return to the porter. The biggest test was opening the door and walking through the crowd of boys.

The expression on my face was scrutinised minutely. A moist eye or the slightest hint of a pained expression would earn me nothing but ridicule. A light step and a confident smile, as if I had received a prestigious prize instead of a severe beating, commanded respect and awe. I had to show complete self-control in the face of pain, which was a struggle, but I dare say it laid the foundations for the resolve I would need to call upon in order to turn my life around in later years.

That evening I contorted myself in front of a mirror. There, I inspected the bright red weals that resembled earthworms on my tender white backside. The strokes were parallel but about an inch apart. It suggested a lack of accuracy, and gave me welcome opportunity to regard the beating skills of my master with utter disdain. I experienced discomfort sitting down for three days, but in my heart I felt as if I had come through a rite of passage with my honour intact.

Following this episode, my relationship with the master greatly improved. He treated me with a certain respect and I no longer caused a problem in the class. Not that one at any rate. A different master delivered my second encounter with the cane, which I inevitably deserved for my attempts to pull focus on myself as he tried to teach. Once again, the marks on my backside were wide enough apart for me to dismiss them as the work of an amateur, and so I lived to disrupt another school day.

The third beating was very different, and really rather extraordinary. We had been given a substitute master whom we had never seen before. We had also been placed in a different classroom, which simply fuelled our high spirits. Our class had a reputation for being unruly and the inexperienced teacher was very nervous. In fact, in order to calm himself and impress his authority upon us, he had already procured the cane and placed it in full view on the top of his desk. Despite this, his hesitant manner, along with the sight of the cane, made us realise he was not in full control. This was a heaven-sent opportunity to create hell.

We were, of course, a nightmare, and I personally took great delight in teasing him mercilessly. Eventually, his patience evaporated. Rather than give due warning, however, the man lost his self-control in the blink of an eye. He drew breath, livid with wrath, and turned two baleful eyes upon me.

'Eugster!' he snapped at me. 'Come here this instant!'

I rose from my desk without breaking from his gaze. I considered myself to be a veteran of the cane by then. I knew that a truly masterful delivery required a level of cool composure. Despite having been on the receiving end of such a punishment twice, I didn't consider either of them to have been delivered effectively. Looking at the man spitting flecks of fury at me, I doubted he would be capable of any precision.

Trembling with rage, and without ordering the other boys to leave, the substitute master grabbed the cane and ordered me to bend over. He then proceeded to strike my behind numerous times and with all the strength he could muster. It hurt, of course, but that was countered by a sense of satisfaction. For his execution lacked any thought. He was simply out of control. It might have spared me the full force of his punishment, but even then my appreciation of technique was something that I would come to value in many other walks of my life. Just as I thought he might continue to blindly thrash me, the master suddenly wheeled away. He was panting for breath and could hardly stand. In response, despite the stinging pain of his assault, I turned around, lifted my chin and smiled at him. I had won, and he knew it.

While corporal punishment was intended to instil discipline and cool hot heads, it didn't have the same impact on me as sport. At St Paul's, I found a host of opportunities to get active. At the same time, I discovered a pursuit that would become a lifelong passion.

Fittingly, rowing played a central role at a school so close to the Thames. As a boy, the chance to join in proved irresistible to me. While I had made my presence known in class by being disruptive, I had hardly shone academically. In fact, one master was moved to say that if my brain were to be placed inside the skull of a sparrow it would rattle!

If I couldn't come alive with an ink pen in hand, I decided, I would do so with an oar instead.

I began rowing in an eight, which reflects the number of oarsmen in the boat. We had four crews in total. I started out at the bottom of the pack, and set about working my way through the ranks. Almost immediately, I found a sense of calm upon the water, and a connection with nature I hadn't registered before. Training early in the morning, with the boat cutting through veils of mist with metronomic grace, I saw all kinds of wildlife on the water that I would otherwise have missed while sleeping in my bed. It was an honour and a pleasure, but it wasn't until I reached the second crew that an episode brought home exactly why rowing was so important to me.

Technique, as I had learned from my punishments and then out on the water, was key to good delivery. A crew is required to work in absolute harmony in order to achieve maximum speed and efficiency. Unless every member is in complete unison with the others, the slightest distraction can undermine the whole exercise. Practice is key, especially ahead of a competition. On one occasion, we were lined up in an amateur regatta against a team of adults from the Thames Rowing Club. I have no idea who thought it would be wise to match boys against men, but we were determined to do our best. It was an intimidating prospect, and so we decided that our best chance would be for the cox to determine when we should put on a spurt based on how the race evolved.

The problem, we discovered, was that the cox had lost his voice. He'd arrived for the event with a heavy cold, and we could barely hear him. So, instead, it fell to one of my fellow rowers at stroke to call the shots.

At the start line, we set off as predicted. The boat crewed by adults pulled away with ease. All we could do was manage the gap, maintain a steady rhythm and await the signal to throw everything at it.

Only the signal never came.

Whether the appointed boy was biding his time or had simply forgotten, he didn't once draw breath to give the signal. By then, the situation was becoming quite desperate. Our competitors continued to pull ahead as we entered a stretch of the river flanked by overgrowth. As the sound of our oars slicing in and out of the water became all the more intense, I just knew that if we didn't go for it in the seconds that followed we would run out of river to catch them.

It was a thought, as if triggered by instinct, that every single member of my crew appeared to experience at that same moment. For as I drew breath, unable to wait any longer, so too did all the other boys, including the oarsman who had taken over the role of cox, and together we yelled: '*Now!*'

At once, we began to pull with all our might. Not only that, the noise of eight young men shouting in a split second at the top of their voices was so deafening that some of the opposing crew stopped rowing. It created chaos in their boat, and their impressive rhythm went awry.

By the time we emerged from the stretch between the overgrown banks, the spectators were presented with the arresting sight of a team of schoolboys leading the way. We crossed the finish line in victorious fashion, leaving our rivals to follow in our wake looking very shamefaced indeed. They sloped off soon afterwards, while I was left in no doubt that the key to being a player in any team sport is *concentration*. You're no longer an individual, but one part of a machine. I cannot explain how we all knew the precise moment to shift gear, but we executed it as a single entity. In a sense it was a humbling lesson, but one also marked by sheer elation. We had defeated a crew of grown men who were too ashamed to admit they had been beaten by a shout. As we didn't admit what had occurred out there on the water, a secret was born between the teams. At school, we were treated like heroes, which was a thrill and an honour. As would always be the case throughout my long life, however, I wasn't content to simply rest upon my laurels.

3

The Button

In 1938, Howard Hughes flew around the world in three days and nineteen hours, the RMS *Queen Elizabeth* embarked on her maiden voyage and Hitler marched into Austria.

Appeasement was in the air, but the fact is that life in London went on as normal. Nobody had any idea that the gathering storm would break with such ferocity and devastation. Like everyone else, my father watched the footage of the German leader ranting madly. While most were simply bemused, he took a more sober view. This was largely down to the fact that he also tuned his shortwave radio into a Swiss station that kept him informed of news and political insight from home.

There, the situation in neighbouring Austria had provoked a greater sense of alarm. This was reflected in each broadcast, which my father followed closely. While he shared his concerns for the welfare of the world with us, I focused on matters that had become all-consuming at the time thanks to my adolescent hormones.

Picking fights in school corridors hadn't got me far, but I remained eager to use my fists. I even wonder whether I had some kind of aggression disorder. Fortunately, sport had become a channel for me to let off steam, to earn some recognition, respect, and – to compensate for my lack of academic skills – even coveted school colours for my achievements. While rowing didn't tolerate physical contact in any shape or form, boxing became increasingly important to me. Having laced up a pair of gloves at such a young age at the Froebel Institute, I found the ring provided both a familiar and an acceptable outlet for my need to land a punch.

Representing St Paul's as a boxer was a great honour. I had once read between the lines of an article in the *Daily Mirror* that reported on the killing of a young man by an ex-pupil of the school. The story told how an argument had developed between the pair outside a nightclub over who had rights to a waiting taxi. The

Old Pauline (a name for the school's alumni that is still used today) struck the other man with one punch. His head hit the kerb, killing him immediately, and the Old Pauline was charged with manslaughter. While the incident was tragic, I couldn't help but note that the accused had once been a member of the first boxing string at the school.

I was taught how to perform in the ring by Mr Begley, a former Empire boxing champion with cauliflower ears after years of pounding. Mr Driscoll, an army instructor, and his father, a seasoned veteran of the sport in his seventieth year, assisted him. Between this trio, I learned to channel my energy with great effect.

As a result of my abilities, I often boxed against opponents from a category above my weight. I had a choice in the matter, but always took up the challenge. Why? Because I felt that being humbled by an equal opponent would be unacceptable to me. I didn't mind losing, so long as the odds were stacked against me from the first bell. By extension, that made a win all the more significant.

In training, Begley and co. taught me the importance of the *button*. This is a term used to describe a point – the size of a £1 coin – close to the tip of the jaw. Hitting this spot hard, so they told me, was a sure-fire way to drop an opponent to the floor, with immediate loss of consciousness. It was an enticing invitation but hard to pull off, as a good fighter will not only keep his chin close to his chest but continuously bob and weave.

I was a tough and determined boxer, and quickly developed a taste for victory. I was also one of those fighters who let his guard down on just one occasion and learned a sobering lesson from the experience. I was fighting in an inter-school bout in Eastbourne. My opponent was the captain of their first boxing team and I was only a second–string contender. To my great delight, as well as that of those who had travelled to watch, I knocked him dizzy in the first round with a well-placed punch. Then, forgetting one vital piece of advice that Begley had taught me, I stood back to let my opponent gather his wits. In response, and possibly gratitude, he recovered to beat my face into a swollen mass and I lost the bout.

My eyes were reduced to narrow slits, my nose pulped and my lips swollen and split. Nothing like this had ever happened to me before. I was destroyed in every way. On my return home later that night, I was terrified that my father would take one look at me and ban me from boxing altogether. Fortunately, he was asleep by the time I crept in, and the swelling reduced overnight so I resembled something partially human at breakfast. It meant I lived to fight another day, and I resolved that I would return to the ring stronger for the experience.

Sure enough, at my next fixture, I gained an advantage early in the second round against a larger opponent. This time, I didn't stand back and give him a chance to recover. Intent on seizing the opportunity, I went straight for the button and left him out cold on the canvas.

My second knockout occurred under less noble circumstances. Instead of a vest and gloves, I was dressed in my Boy Scout uniform. We were taking part in an after-dark exercise with another Scout group from London, and had gathered at a church hall in their neighbourhood. The host troop's scoutmaster had issued us with a most bizarre task. In pairs, we were expected to head out under the stars and return with three specific items: a copy of the *Daily Mail* from the previous day, a lady's bra and a black cat. It was patently ridiculous, and designed, I suspect, for us to fail. Still, we took up the challenge with the utmost seriousness. Naturally, our group had no idea where to begin. We'd creep into back yards and find nothing. Meanwhile the other Scout group members simply scurried home to pick up pets, rifle through their mother's underwear drawer and grab a discarded newspaper on the way back out. Unsurprisingly, unlike those boys, we returned with nothing to show for ourselves.

It was a hollow victory, I thought, and left a sour taste in my mouth for the rest of the evening. We finished with a simple but rowdy game of tag in which our group were tasked with reaching the church hall while our opponents attempted to grab a length of wool that each of us had been instructed to tie on to our left arm. We were ambushed, of course, but I was determined that nobody would catch me. After some deft manoeuvring in the moonlight shadows I seized my chance to dash for the church doors. A cry went up straight away, and I found myself sprinting along the path under the stars with Boy Scouts on their home turf baying behind me. Just as I thought I would make it, the scoutmaster stepped into my field of vision. Grinning, he spread his hands wide to stop me. He also made the mistake of tipping his chin into the moonlight. Instinctively, and without compromise, I drew my fist back and smacked him. For once, my punch landed squarely on the button! I didn't even see him go down. I just hurtled for the door with a victorious cry.

I waited inside for a moment, expecting the Scouts from the other group to follow behind and congratulate me. When nobody joined me inside the doors, I stepped back out onto the path to find them crowding warily around their fallen leader. A bush had broken his fall, but not softened the injury to his pride. I was, of course, severely reprimanded for what was deemed 'a vicious attack'. In truth, having been sent on a wild goose chase by the man, I can only look back at the moment I landed that punch and confess that I'd enjoyed it.

While I had a talent for boxing to rival my passion for rugby and rowing, my interest in girls at that time failed to bring me any kind of success. For the boys of St Paul's, perhaps the most important event of 1938 was the first annual dance with pupils from nearby St Paul's Girls' School. In preparation, the Great Hall was cleared and the floor polished for dancing. While our masters were present to oversee the event, so too were their wives. As a result, the dance was important to me for two distinct reasons. First, it meant there was a possibility that by meeting the masters' wives I could glean information concerning their private lives that might prove useful. Second, I had a desperate need to meet a girl who could relieve me of my virginity.

Those boys who claimed to have been intimate with the opposite sex were in an extremely small minority. Even so, they were regarded with awe and admiration. They were also a valuable source of advice. I learned that entering into a relationship with a virgin should be avoided at all costs. It wasn't just down to the lack of experience on their part, they said. Apparently a virgin would never, *ever* let you break up with her. This meant I had to find a girl who was both sophisticated and experienced. I just didn't know how to begin finding one, because asking directly was out of the question. Even if I did strike lucky, their clothes presented enormous difficulties. Female undergarments such as bloomers or cami-knickers were frustrating and formidable barriers. But these were nothing compared to girdles or corsets that required all the ingenuity of the cleverest human being to circumvent. Or so I had been told, at least.

In a bid to bolster my confidence, I borrowed my father's dinner jacket, dress shirt and wing collar. As the advertisements of the day told me that if I used Brylcreem on my hair I would be more attractive to women, I plastered my hair with the stuff. My hair turned into a bright shiny mass. On setting off for the dance, it actually felt as if I was wearing a tight skull-cap. I was ready!

In the Great Hall, practically all the boys sported dinner jackets, while the girls wore long evening gowns. It was a lively and festive affair with an orchestra providing the music. The popular songs at the time included 'September Song' and 'Falling In Love With Love', and the floor quickly filled. I stood on the sidelines for a while, hoping to tick off one of my objectives for the evening by talking to the wife of one of my rowing teachers. During the course of our conversation, she told me that she always knew when our crew had suffered a bad outing as her husband would come home grumpy. As intelligence gathering went, I could have done better. Still, it meant I would go on to feel a bit sad for her whenever we performed badly in regattas.

As the evening progressed, I turned my attention to my second goal. My spirits rose considerably on finding a girl who agreed to dance with me. After treading on her toes for a couple of numbers, I persuaded her to sneak outside with me and sit on the bench in the dark to look at the moon. A period of passionate necking followed, but not for long as we were both scared of being discovered. We hurried back inside as if nothing had happened, only to look at each other in horror on crossing the lighted threshold. Where I had stepped outside with a beauty, I now faced a girl with a face smeared in make-up and Brylcreem. That most of it was all over my face and my father's shirt and his dinner jacket, I went on to discover, made things even worse. Aghast, we rushed to our respective restrooms, and there I scrubbed desperately at myself in a bid to look half respectable. Eventually, I admitted defeat and scurried home before anyone spotted me.

I considered that evening to be an unmitigated disaster. Some time later, St Paul's Girls' School hosted a dance for us, and that's when things went from really bad to even worse.

Wearing a dinner jacket my mother had purchased just for me, presumably because she didn't wish to risk me ruining another one belonging to my father, I arrived with my expectations lowered considerably. This time I was determined to find a girl who hadn't bothered with make-up, and didn't care whether she was sophisticated or experienced. As luck would have it, I found a young lady who actually fitted the bill. After a few dances, she even offered to show me around the school. Having led me down several corridors, she stopped in front of a nondescript door.

'This is a very special room,' she told me with a twinkle in her eye, and indeed it was extraordinary. On opening the door for me, she invited me to inspect a space with padding on the walls and ceiling.

'What happens in here?' I asked.

The girl responded by clicking the door shut behind her.

'It's a music room,' she purred. 'I practise my cello in here.'

She went on to describe how wide she had to open her legs to accommodate the instrument. It seemed like an unnecessary detail to me. I simply responded by looking up and around.

'So, this is soundproofed?' I observed.

'Completely,' she said, waiting until she had my full attention. 'If someone were to scream out loud in here,' she added, and knocked me a wink, 'nobody would know.'

I frowned, perplexed by her line of conversation. 'Right,' I said, feeling a little uncomfortable all of a sudden, and made my way back out into the corridor. 'Well, thank you for the tour!'

Half an hour later, while dancing with another girl, the significance of what my guide had said suddenly dawned on me! Having spent years being told by teachers that I wasn't up to much academically, here was evidence to prove that I was in fact *completely stupid*. An attractive girl had offered to extract my virginity, and I'd responded by politely taking my leave.

I spent the rest of that evening frantically searching for the girl, but to no avail. I was devastated, plagued by nightmares that she might have found another boy who could satisfy her desires, but also determined not to feel this way again. When faced with an opportunity, I resolved, whether it concerned the opposite sex who showed an interest in me or any other aspect of my life, I would do my utmost not to let it slip through my fingers.

4

The Grand Crew in Ostend

Towards the end of my time at St Paul's, at the tail end of 1938, talk turned to the possibility that we really might go to war with Germany.

Rumours often swept through the capital as much as the school corridors. We heard that barges had been moored along the Thames stocked with coal to burn pyres of human bodies in the wake of an aerial bombardment. When we came into school one morning to find a trench had been dug across the school playing field, in preparation for an invasion, it seemed very real to us all. I enquired why the trenches weren't shored up with timber, and was told that wood might absorb poisons from a chemical attack, and render them toxic for years to come. As I was troop leader in the Boy Scouts, I was made 'Fire Chief' and my troop the school's fire brigade.

It was an unsettling time, with hearsay running rampant. As schoolboys we painted our own picture of what could happen next. While Germany was largely embodied by footage of a ranting Hitler, we had already formed our view of what their soldiers looked like. This followed a visit from a German school that had taken place several terms earlier. At a time of appeasement, it was believed that talking to one another would somehow avert conflict. In practice, it simply reinforced our perception of the enemy we faced.

The group had arrived accompanied by a teacher and an official from the Nazi party. Due to lack of foreign exchange such overseas travel was a huge privilege for these boys, who regarded themselves as 'the master race'. Most were blond with close-cropped hair and maintained a military posture at all times. I never once saw them with their hands in their pockets (which was for them forbidden). Most striking of all, perhaps, was the fact that they oozed self-confidence and vitality. By contrast, while they were dressed in smart grey suits, my friends and I slouched around with canteen food stains on our lapels.

Our visitors regarded us with quiet disdain. We must have represented everything they'd been warned about back home. Through their eyes, degenerates populated England, and the only thing that could bring them into line was German discipline and order. What they hadn't been told by their masters – and it had quite possibly been withheld from them – was the fact that St Paul's boasted an Officers' Training Corps run by the Coldstream Guards. As a public school, the focus of our education at that time was to administer, defend or even expand the Empire. Learning to shoot with ordnance rifles was compulsory, while an emphasis on team sports encouraged us to push at our physical and mental limits. Overall, it was a cold and formal encounter, as they could not speak English and the Nazi official and their master never let them out of sight. They later visited Oxford, which was to become the capital of England after London had been destroyed according to Nazi plans. Even so, it was an encounter that would go on to linger in our minds as we sailed towards adulthood and the brink of war.

Despite enjoying my time at the school, I left St Paul's feeling as if very few of my ambitions had been realised. Academically, I had learned to scrape through every exam with the least amount of work possible. I fared better in sport, achieving colours in rowing (1st

VIII), rugby (2nd XV) and boxing (2nd String), and yet I departed as a virgin. In my book, I considered this to be a broken dream.

It would be some time before that burden was lifted, and I discovered that life didn't change one bit as a result. Until then, it felt like a burden I was destined to continue shouldering. This was made just a little easier to bear on obtaining a place at Guy's Hospital to study dentistry. In view of my questionable academic prowess, however, I remain convinced that there must have been some mistake in the selection process.

My reason for choosing a career as a dentist was very simple. I had always admired physicians for their work. My grandfather had taken the Hippocratic Oath, in fact. I was also mindful of the fact that he had once observed that being a doctor was 'a dog's life' which didn't hold much appeal. In particular, he claimed his profession prevented him from having holidays, and he even forbade my father from following in his footsteps. Unwilling to dedicate myself to such a degree, and aware of my mental shortcomings, I decided that dentistry would bring me the same gravitas as medicine but with less effort and more leisure time. Rather than studying the entire body, I would be restricted to a set number of teeth, and so I embarked upon a course of study that would one day be interrupted by world events. Until that moment arrived, I sought to keep up with my fellow students as best I could, while hoping my tutors didn't have second thoughts about me.

As a student at Guy's, I joined the Thames Rowing Club. Unlike my studies, I could commit myself to a sporting endeavour and duly shine for my efforts. I had the honour of competing in the Henley Royal Regatta and then, in 1939, received an invitation to compete internationally in the Belgian coastal city of Ostend. What made the prospect even more exciting was the fact that our crew were set to race a representation from Germany.

The war had yet to begin, but by then we knew our enemy.

Much like the visiting school party who had considered us to be beneath them, we found the German rowing team to be equally distant and aloof. We were all aware of the Nazi propaganda that boasted of their racial superiority. The way the crew regarded themselves when we arrived ahead of the race, it felt as if we were up against superhumans who were simply there to pick up the winners' medals. They had been carefully selected, which made us all the more determined to put them in their place.

We weren't alone in wanting to beat them. Just

before our practice outing, a number of Belgians approached us.

'*Je vous en prie, il faut que vous battiez les allemandes,*' they said politely, speaking low as if fearful of being overheard.

In my best French, I promised them that we would indeed do our level best to win, and I meant every word. We hadn't simply come here to compete. In view of what was happening in Europe, we had to beat the Germans at all costs.

Often in a situation like this, the battle is as psychological as it is physical, and here we found an early advantage. It wasn't something that we could have planned. In fact, until it happened I had no idea that an object as simple as butter could rattle our opponents.

Unknown to us, as part of the Nazi campaign to prepare the German public for war, restrictions had been placed on certain items in order to boost military funding. Butter was on the list of prohibited items. I later learned that they even promoted a slogan: '*Kanonen statt Butter*', which translated as 'guns instead of butter'. A patriotic German, therefore, would make such a sacrifice without question, and that extended to ventures overseas.

On the eve of the race, the German crew had reserved a table in an exclusive restaurant in Ostend.

Aware of the restrictions, but assuming the visiting crew would turn a blind eye so far from home, the maître d' informed the captain that the chef made full use of all ingredients ... including certain dairy produce. '*Nous avons une cuisine de beurre,*' he told him discreetly.

In response, well aware of what this meant, the captain grew red in the face. He then yelled in German, dressing down the poor man and his staff, before snapping into a Nazi salute and turning on his heels. The Germans marched out, making it quite clear that in being offered butter they had just endured a grave insult. At the same time, they left the maître d' feeling equally affronted. Even today, if you want to upset a Belgian or a Frenchman, all you have to do is to pour scorn on their cuisine.

The news spread across town quickly. It reached us as we enjoyed a very fine supper indeed that most probably had been cooked in lavish amounts of butter. The Belgians were deeply offended by the behaviour of the German party, and many went home at the end of the evening muttering darkly about revenge.

The next morning, as the sun rose over the canal that would host our race, several locals approached us. This time, they conveyed their request as if something more important than money was resting on the outcome. They also made no effort to keep their voices down. 'Sirs,' they said in their native tongue, though the sentiment needed no translation. '*You must beat the bastards!*'

With the weight of expectation on our shoulders, I gathered with the crew to talk through our strategy.

'The start signal is *Êtes-vous prêts?* (Are you ready?) *Parti!* (Go!)' our stroke informed us. 'If we go on "*prêts*",' he suggested, 'we'll seize an advantage.'

I glanced at my teammates with some uncertainty. We could easily claim that the signal had been lost in translation, someone argued. In fact, even though it would give us a chance to sink our oars into the water ahead of our rivals the advantage had to be so slight that people would be unlikely to notice.

On that basis, well aware that the pride of a nation was at stake, we agreed to reinterpret the rules in our favour.

We rowed up the canal to the start to find that masses of people had gathered at the banks. They stood in deathly silence. Behind them, spectators crammed the frames of almost every window of the water-front houses. Without a word, we drew alongside the German boat. Neither team even glanced at the other. There, for what felt like an eternity, we awaited the start signal.

And when it came, we knew exactly what we had to do.

'*Êtes . . . vous . . . prêts?*'

On that third word we sprang into action.

'*Parti!*'

After several strokes, pulling with all my might, I dared to look for the other boat. I expected to see them fighting to catch up, but they were nowhere to be seen! Then I heard their cox, bellowing instruction in German, and realised they were ahead of us. There could be only one explanation. Before launching, our rivals hadn't even waited for the word *prêts*.

Not only had they stolen an advantage greater than the one that we had pilfered, their lane was in better water. Protected from the wind by the trees on the bank at this side, they began to increase the gap between us.

At 500 metres we were two lengths down. We had blown it, and I knew from experience that every single member of my crew was thinking exactly the same thing. Without instruction, we simply threw everything we had at rowing our best. Defeat seemed almost inevitable, and yet we had to show that we had put our heart and soul into the endeavour. It all came down to technique, and indeed there was a moment when we were rowing in perfect synchronicity. This is a rare thing in rowing, but when it happens the feeling is one of both calm and sheer elation.

At the same time, a little further ahead, the Germans cleared the windbreak of trees and rowed into the same choppy water as us. This put us on an equal footing, and yet we'd had several seconds to fine-tune our engine. From that moment on, with every pull of our oars, we began to catch our quarry.

The roar from the onlookers was intense. Every single Belgian on the banks and at the windows was urging us to catch them. By now, we had come so close to our rivals we could hear every grunt and exhalation. We drew level with the German boat just as the finish came into view, and then finally beat them by half a length.

As the prow of our boat crossed the line, it seemed as if the whole of Ostend erupted.

That evening, we were treated as heroes. People flocked to shake our hands and congratulate *les anglais*, and both beer and champagne flowed. I must confess things became a little rowdy as we visited one bar after another. I became scared and attached myself to a thirteen-stone member of the crew called O'Mara. We visited an exclusive restaurant to be greeted with applause. A gentleman who was with his mistress asked us how we managed to win. O'Mara swept all the glasses, plates, food and everything else on the table to the floor. He then sat on the table in front of the gentleman and his petrified mistress to demonstrate our style of rowing. I managed to get him out of the restaurant, fearing a huge bill for damages, but everyone just cheered. I'm not entirely clear what happened after that as I subsequently blacked out. I simply have to assume that my larger-than-life companion saw me back to our hotel safely.

The next morning, nursing torturous headaches, we were summoned to the town hall. There, despite worries that we might be facing some kind of admonishment for our behaviour, we were presented with our victory prize. One by one, and with genuine gratitude, the mayor handed out medals. To our surprise, as no oarsman would ever smoke, he also gifted us each a gold-plated Ronson lighter. In those days such a prestigious item was regarded as tool for seduction in the right hands. If you could light a lady's cigarette with a Ronson, so it was said, then she would without fail be unable to resist your charms. On returning home, it would be some time before I put the theory into practice. In some part, this was down to the fact that my hangover lasted more than two weeks.

Some time later, thankfully unshackled from the chains of my virginity, I met a very attractive young lady and spent the night with her. With only a little experience under my belt, I was so overwhelmed by her amazing skills in bed that I felt I must show my appreciation. So I gave her my prized Ronson lighter, to my everlasting regret, as she then vanished from my life altogether. Looking back at this whole episode, which was in effect our last moment of high spirits before war broke out, I learned three vital lessons:

Lesson 1: A race is never over until the last stroke.

Lesson 2: Never mix beer with champagne.

Lesson 3: Never, *ever*, give away your prizes!

5

A Sacrifice for the Common Good

'What do you see, Eugster?'

My examiner at Guy's had invited me to inspect the contents of a glass jar. I found myself looking at something fleshy and unpleasant suspended in a liquid inside.

'Is it a piece of meat?' I offered, with no clue to its identity. I watched the man's expression draw tight with indignation.

'A piece of *meat*?' he repeated, as if barely able to comprehend the depths of my idiocy as an aspiring dentist. 'It's a human tongue with cancer!'

I had reached the end of my first year studying at Guy's. My heroic return from the rowing duel in

Ostend was in the past, Britain was on the brink of mobilisation, and I faced the very real possibility of being drummed out of dentistry. As ever, I had put in the least amount of study possible. Following my encounter with the tongue in a jar, and having chalked up several basic errors preceding this, I paid the price by failing one critical discipline. There was no way, I believed, that I would be permitted to continue my studies the following academic year.

Then again, I never suffered the indignity of being asked to leave because war got in the way. One day, I returned home from Guy's to discover my father packing up our belongings in preparation for a hasty move to Switzerland. While an air of uncertainty continued to weigh over London, my father had heard quite enough about Hitler's intentions from dialling into the radio broadcasts from his homeland. My mother, by then, was chronically incapacitated by illness and morphine addiction. If the capital was to come under attack, and he was convinced that this would happen without notice, then it was no place to be caring for his invalid wife.

Such was my father's concern that he gave me no choice in the matter. And so we set off for a country that I had often visited on holiday as a boy, and which would eventually become my lifelong home.

Switzerland, during the war, remained neutral. While no fighting took place inside her borders, this country of four million citizens boasted a large army that operated under rules of conscription. Having arrived in Zurich with my parents, and being of Swiss nationality, I was duly called up to join 400,000 men. I passed a rigorous medical, which left my muscles sore for weeks, before joining an infantry that contained several fellow countrymen who had also lived abroad. Interestingly, one chap was from Germany. He had simply crossed the border before the war, seeking to buy wallpaper for his company back home, and ended up pitted against his home country. An old Russian of Swiss nationality also numbered in our ranks, as reliable as he was resentful at his situation, which rendered us a curious band of brothers overall.

My experience of the training process was governed by hunger, which was a horrible experience. This was down to the fact that our commanding officer wished to take us to warmer climes to the south of the country, but didn't possess the funds to travel. In order to save money, he cut back on our rations. We survived on bread made with potatoes, which had a stringy quality. It would always be served at lunchtimes with polenta and one drop of meat sauce. When we finally made it south we were billeted in a small village. There, the inhabitants were so shocked at the way we were treated that they physically attacked our officers. It was a gruelling and deeply testing time. Every now and then, I would receive a package from my father that contained salami. Without this, I believe I might have starved. I looked forward to receiving such packages, and catching up with news from Zurich. Until one day I received the devastating news that my mother had passed away. Her health had deteriorated significantly since the move to Switzerland, which finally saw her tragic life cut short.

I might have been skin and bone when I saw my father again, but to my eyes he had changed more dramatically than me, for his hair had turned completely white. By all accounts it had gone that way over the course of just ten days. He suffered the loss very badly, and after I returned to my regiment I learned that he had decided to go back to London. There were no hostilities during that period, which was known as 'the phoney war'. The expected bombing raids had failed to materialise. Heartbroken, and possibly wishing to haunt a place that reminded him of a happier time with his young wife, I can only think he believed it would be safe. I applied for foreign leave in order to join him, only for the Germans to begin their offensive. Duly I returned to my unit just a short time before London endured the Blitz, unaware that I would never see him again.

Serving in a neutral country during wartime is a curious mix of internal military manoeuvres and a semblance of normality. The Swiss army system permitted long periods of leave, even throughout the war years. In effect, I would find myself in a cycle of being discharged and then called up again. So I used my free time to enrol at university in Zurich in order to salvage my desire to become a dentist. The study requirements were very different. After failing and then finally passing some strange exams to support my application I found myself back on track. I also picked up the oars once more and joined a rowing club. Like Thames, this one boasted a notable reputation, having won the Stewards, the Grand and the Diamonds at Henley and two medals at the Olympics. I would have to drop everything whenever the next call-up came, of course, but that soon became a way of life for me. During my time in military uniform, I should say, I never once fired my weapon in battle. It was as a civilian that I saw action. Just not in the conventional sense.

During a period at the university in Zurich, a Dutch student called Bill befriended me. He had travelled to Switzerland to study but fallen on hard times. His parents had been Dutch diplomats in Sumatra, and after Japan invaded Indonesia nothing was ever heard from them again. It left Bill with no financial support, and in a bid to survive he had offered his services to the American Secret Service in Switzerland. When he proved himself to be a trusted operative, the US agency commissioned Bill to run a covert operation in the south of the country. Having got to know each other well, he approached me for help.

'Can you cook?' he enquired one day.

'Of course!' I declared, almost offended that he'd had to ask. 'In the Boy Scouts we learned to prepare food over an open fire. We even had to eat it!'

Bill laughed, and quietly explained what would be required. In Zurich at the time, food rationing was severe. Hungry and with an appetite for adventure, I accepted the invitation.

Soon afterwards, we travelled to Ticino, a region of forested valleys and lakes bordering northern Italy. Here, Bill took me to a large villa in Lugano, in the southern part of Switzerland, where he informed me that I would be preparing meals for between six and ten people. Knowing Bill's connection with the US Secret Service, and their commitment to supporting the Allies, I chose not to ask further questions. In some ways, there was no need. As soon as the guests began to arrive, I worked out what was going on.

Just over the border, the Italian Fascists were struggling to contain the resistance movement. When men with hunted expressions began to arrive, dressed in civilian clothing, I knew they belonged to the Italian or Yugoslavian partisan movement.

Over the course of their stay, with my assumptions proven correct, this band of resistance fighters quickly came to trust me. They had been invited here to rest as well as to share intelligence and hatch plans, and I did my level best to make sure that they were well fed. They stayed for about a week before disappearing, only for another group to arrive. As the operation was at odds with Switzerland's neutral role, I was careful to keep my mouth shut when shopping for provisions in the nearby village. Here, non-rationed food could be bought that had been smuggled from Italy. Bill knew that he could trust me in this. The focus for his misgivings, I learned, rested with the villa's landlady. Bill had given her a cover story when he rented it, but now he feared that she had noted the activity and suspected what was really going on.

'We have to shut her up in case she talks,' he told me, which sounded ominous.

'How?' I asked, trying not to sound alarmed.

Bill appraised me carefully. 'Charles, we all need to make sacrifices for the common good at this time.'

'I suppose so.'

'You're a handsome sort of chap,' he went on, 'and, well . . . we believe with some gentle persuasion she might fall for your charms.'

Slowly, the penny dropped. 'You want me to . . .'

My voice trailed away as Bill began to nod like I had no choice in the matter.

The next day, reminding myself that I was doing this for a greater purpose, I invited the villa's land-lady out to dinner. As I was one of the rental party, she regarded me cautiously at first. Finally, once I'd persisted as warmly as I could, she relented and agreed. Bill hadn't spelled out exactly what was required. I had no clear strategy, but told myself that if I had to take her to bed then I would do exactly that. It didn't help that the poor woman was far from my type. I also worried that I might not be her cup of tea, which would mean failing in my mission in the worst possible way. All I could do was wine and dine her to the best of my abilities. As the evening progressed, however, I actually came to enjoy her company and she certainly warmed to me. I can only think my efforts drained her energies, however, because at the end of our date she bid me goodnight with a happy smile, which saved me from taking things further.

The next time I saw Bill, he chose not to debrief me in detail. He simply told me that whatever went on between the landlady and me must have worked wonders, because ever since her misgivings about the continuous comings and goings had vanished. Later, when the partisans had been smuggled back over the border to continue their operations against the Nazis, my friend thanked me for my efforts in the kitchen and beyond. It was, without doubt, an exciting, testing but enlightening experience. Even though I later learned that the Swiss Secret Service were wise to it, and had quietly allowed it to take place, I left feeling like I had made a small but not insignificant contribution to the war effort. We were part of the operation 'Sunrise' to persuade the German General Wolff in Italy to surrender.

Periods of military service followed, which proved free of action and espionage, as well as light on food. After each stint, I would head straight to Zurich to push on with my studies. The war had turned my efforts to train as a dentist into a protracted affair. Even as the years began to tick by, however, I was determined to see it through. I stayed with relatives of my father each time I went back, but saw little of them. Instead, in a

55

bid to make the most of my opportunities away from the regiment, I would get up at the crack of dawn and then cycle the long journey to university for a day of lectures (which started at 7.15 a.m.) and practical lessons. Afterwards, as evening approached, I would pedal to the lake for an hour of rowing on the water. By the time I returned to my relatives it was too late for supper, and so I would retire to repeat the routine the next day. It left me tired, hungry and frequently chilled to the bone, but I didn't complain. Even when a feverish patient coughed into my face during a practical training session in my final year, I simply got on with the task in hand.

A short time later, I was diagnosed with tuberculosis. In effect, I had worn down my immune system through a combination of undernourishment and strenuous exercise. As a result, discharged from the army for being medically unfit, I spent six months cooped up in a Swiss sanatorium. Most of that time I spent being very cross with myself for being so stupid.

My stay coincided with the end of the war. Afterwards, I returned to Zurich to complete my studies. Finally, with the usual minimal pass marks, I qualified to practise as a dentist in the country. Having risked everything by showing no regard for my health, however, I was determined to learn from the experience. I may have lapsed several times in the many decades that followed, but I now consider that newfound outlook to be the bedrock of successful ageing. The key, I would go on to discover, was in the science of maintaining that foundation.

6

Platinum, Gold . . . and Dollars

I marked the end of the war, along with my return to health, by leaving Zurich and heading back to London. As well as needing to take care of my father's affairs – he had been bombed out and died while I was in Switzerland – I was keen to see if I could resume my studies at Guy's. I had qualified to practise dentistry in Switzerland, but in my opinion it didn't match the quality of learning available in one of the most prestigious medical schools in the world.

The question was whether they would be prepared to have me back.

Not only did I have a dismal academic performance on record at the hospital, the competition for entry was intense. In the wake of demobilisation, soldiers were given stipends and grants to study. Those who had put their medical careers on hold flocked to the capital in a bid to secure a place on the course. Yes, I had a dental diploma from the University of Zurich that proved I wasn't a complete flop, but from the moment I arrived at the interview it seemed that the odds were stacked against me.

'Tell us, Candidate Eugster, how many years did you serve in the Swiss army?'

The question from the panel caused me to pause. Before me, seated at a table on a raised platform, ten academics waited as I attempted to cobble together my numerous call-ups.

'It's calculated by the number of days rather than months or years,' I offered weakly, before trying and failing to convert the figures into an acceptable answer.

Things did not look good. Then, at the left of the platform, the professor who had been studying my old dossier broke into a smile and passed it on. In turn, the panel's expressions brightened, and to my amazement they offered me a place on the course. The reason was most unexpected, but once again rowing came to my rescue.

At some point before the war, I had competed in

a four against another hospital crew on the Thames. Somehow we won, and this had earned me a 'half blue' and a special tie to wear. Sporting rivalry among the teaching hospitals continued to be intense, and was duly recognised by the panel. As a result, this almost forgotten win came to contribute to my career.

Duly enrolled once more at Guy's, with fortunes brightening in many different ways, I didn't make life any easier for myself. At the time, a young lady had come to augment rowing as a central interest in my life. As I spent more time exploring her anatomy than I did at lectures on the same subject, I duly failed the first part of my final exam. Quietly hoping that my abilities with an oar might compensate for my academic shortcomings, I accepted an invitation to row for the hospital team. As we also had an Oxford Blue in the crew, which in my view made us unbeatable, I hoped that victory on the water might once again smooth waters elsewhere. Unfortunately, my presence in the boat coincided with losing a major competition and a massive silver trophy. Through my eyes, it was inevitable that shortly after that defeat I should receive a letter to inform me that because of my poor academic results, which could not be tolerated, I would be expelled unless I passed a special exam. Rowing had got me back into Guy's, and now it seemed it had nearly got me thrown out. I was left with no choice but to focus hard on my studies.

Finally, through guile as much as graft, I achieved what I had set out to do and graduated from the Royal College of Surgeons. As a qualified dentist, I could now practise in the UK as well as Switzerland. Like all challenges I would take on in life, I hadn't made it easy for myself. Even so, I never gave up, and that made the journey all the more meaningful.

For someone who struggled with exams, which was largely down to minimal effort at coursework and last-minute revision, it may seem surprising to learn that I remained hungry for more. Despite my inherent laziness, I was genuinely interested in the field of dentistry and everything there was to know about the subject. So, having finished with Guy's, I set my sights on a doctorate. This meant writing a thesis, and a journey to Germany that proved to be a complete waste in one respect and an invaluable experience in another.

My impression of the country at that time, such a short while after the war, was one of life among ruins. I travelled to the university at Bonn, which was one of the few buildings that hadn't been bombed out. There, I had hoped to study under the tutelage of an eminent professor. Instead of enjoying his undivided attention so that I might debate the finer points of my thesis, I found they did things very differently compared to my experience in Switzerland and London. There, I discovered that rather than working with just one small group of students, my professor was responsible for a great raft of different subjects across the faculty. As a result, I was expected to wait for several hours until he could see me, only for him to afford me just five minutes of his time. It was hopeless! But then, once he had learned that I intended to focus on gum disease, he declared that a respected professor in Berlin had an interesting theory on the cause. And so I left for the capital. Not just to pursue my damned thesis but out of sheer curiosity.

In 1948, Berlin existed not just under occupation but a blockade. This was an early confrontation in the Cold War, when the Russians squared up to the Allied forces over rail, road and canal access to the German capital. I arrived to find another city picking itself up from the ground, and it seemed to me that the citizens existed in a climate of bureaucracy and paperwork. Rationing remained in force, which meant producing the right documentation in order to survive, while freedom of movement was heavily curtailed by the compartmentalisation of the city into zones. I was lucky, having obtained authorisation to visit as a member of the occupying forces. It meant in due course I could travel to the French zone in order to locate the professor who would help me with my thesis. As for my hotel, I found the building surrounded by ruins, with a doorman on duty wearing white tie and tails! The guests were mostly officers wearing a huge amount of gold braid. The food was excellent with porridge and a full English breakfast plus afternoon tea. Settled in and nourished beyond my expectation, I set out to find the object of my visit.

When I finally tracked down the professor, I learned to my horror that he was in fact completely senile. I have no idea how he managed to remain in his post, because his mental shortcomings were obvious to me within minutes of our meeting. Almost immediately, my hopes and dreams came crashing down. Pursuing my thesis here in Berlin would get me nowhere. Making my excuses, I decided that I should at least get to know the city before abandoning my plans.

Outside, just wandering the streets, I became acutely aware of whispers whenever people passed me by. I began to listen carefully, and soon detected what was being offered to me.

'*Platinum . . . gold . . . dollars.*'

This was a city with a population that resorted to barter in order to stay alive. People were desperate to exchange. They included one young German lady with whom I struck up a conversation. She proved to be both resilient and delightful, and when she invited me to tour the east of the city where she lived, which was under Russian occupation, I jumped at the chance.

On the day of our rendezvous, I hopped on a train that would take me through the checkpoint. Every seat in the carriage was taken. Chatter and laughter filled the air. Then the most extraordinary thing happened. As soon as we crossed from West Berlin to the East, the noise inside the carriage just fell away. Suddenly, nobody said a word. What's more, once I'd disembarked and met my lady friend I found that charged atmosphere extended to the streets. From there on out, as we passed Russian soldiers patrolling the streets, I felt nothing but tension in the air. It was horrible. My lady friend seemed quite used to it, and had clearly learned to survive under those challenging circumstances. I would go on to spend the night at her flat. I didn't have the right papers to remain in the zone overnight, but I considered it a risk worth taking. The next day, on returning to the relative sunshine of the West, I arrived under no illusion that this was a city divided between two forces intent on shaping the wider world. I also knew on which side I wished to be when it came to forging ahead with my life. Just then, however, Berlin no longer held any promise for me. If I wanted to seize the opportunities that lay in wait, I needed to venture much further west.

I arrived in Chicago on the cusp of the 1950s. In terms of culture, industry and communications, the world was evolving at a terrific pace. Having abandoned my hopes of writing my thesis in Germany, I had come here to pursue my studies at the Windy City's Northwestern University in what I hoped would be a more supportive environment. My hunch proved right, while America at the time was an exciting place to be. I loved every moment, and embraced the way of life wholeheartedly.

Following my father's death, and the execution of his estate, I had found myself with a little money in my pocket. He was by no means wealthy at the end, having walked away from work at an early age. Nevertheless, my inheritance enabled me to cross the Atlantic in order to chase the qualifications I wanted so badly, an intention underpinned by a genuine desire to absorb and understand every aspect of my chosen subject. By then, I believe my inclination towards laziness had finally subsided. Alongside that, I found myself in a post-war country that just begged me to travel and explore. So, as I reached the end of my time at Northwestern University, I purchased a black Chevrolet with leather upholstery and white-walled tyres, jumped in and set off for a round trip of the USA. To fund my journey, I turned to stock market speculation.

Rather than see my money go up in smoke, however, it actually worked out in my favour. It covered the cost of my trip without breaking the bank and allowed me to sate my wanderlust. By the time my journey was over, I was ready to embark upon what felt like the next stage in my life. On the road to achieving my doctorate, well travelled and no longer appalled at my lack of experience with women, I headed back to Europe to graduate with a view to starting a business, and even a family.

To begin with, in order to complete my doctorate, I spent some time in Germany once more. In Bonn, during my first visit, I had been struck by how positive the people were in the face of adversity. They seemed to have festivals for all occasions, celebrating everything from petals to wine. I admired this quality greatly, and settled for a while in Heidelberg to finish my studies at the university. I had been profoundly influenced by my time in America, however. Rather than turn my back on her completely, I had traded in my Chevy for an Oldsmobile 98 upholstered in red leather before leaving and arranged to have it shipped to Europe. It was an unusual move, almost unheard of at the time, but it proved to have a profound impact on the direction of my life. This huge, magnificent vehicle effectively followed me to Europe, and ensured that people paid attention whenever I hit the road.

As a man in his early thirties, smartly dressed and cruising around town, it proved to be quite the attraction. I must admit that it was responsible for kick-starting a conversation on the street with an admirer who turned out to be the wife of an economics professor. In due course this led to a friendship and then to something more. Understandably, though I was too blinkered and cocksure to feel bad, the professor was quite devastated. I was far younger than him, in possession of an impressive American car and his wife's undivided attention. Now, rather than square up to me, the poor beleaguered man played a very different game. His first move, in fact, was to invite me to a party.

'I should like you to attend as my guest,' he said. 'It's a faculty event, and all my students will be present. If anyone takes your fancy, just let me know and I will make an introduction.'

Out of curiosity as much as guilt, I accepted his invitation. I'll never know whether he had ensured that the finest young female student on his course would be there to catch my eye. But when I saw her I felt sure that she was the one for me. Her name was Edda Bianca. She had dark hair, fathomless eyes and an enchanting smile. We got along just beautifully, which left the professor both delighted and relieved. In fact, it was a course of events that left everyone happy. The professor's marriage survived my interference, Edda Bianca received outstanding marks from him in her final paper (and I shall always maintain that I played a role in this achievement), and she went on to become my wife.

7

A Lump of Lard

1954 was marked by two significant events in my life. First, Edda Bianca and I got married. Then, having completed my doctorate, and on moving into an apartment in Zurich, I took steps to open my first dental practice. Despite showing a lack of promise in the early days of my education, an ineptitude that extended to women, I had finally arrived at one of life's most significant stages. I was no longer young and carefree, but comfortable with routine and building a sense of security. This, I believe, is where we risk becoming complacent, which is precisely what happened to me.

In establishing a new business, it's inevitable that other interests in life take a back seat. Rowing was still important to me, but demands on my time meant I rarely had a chance to get out on to the lake. I renewed my membership at the club in Zurich, but considered myself to be nothing more than a hobby rower. While Edda Bianca furnished a home for us, I sought premises in the city for my practice that were in keeping with my lofty ambition.

My plan, I had decided on returning to Switzerland, was to cater to a high-end clientele. In very simple terms, it meant I could earn more money from my expertise. The challenge was in setting myself apart from the competition. Every dentist effectively offers the same service, after all. Oral hygiene is important to everyone regardless of their bank balance. So, instead of selling myself on my hard-earned skills, and building a practice that suited me, I set out to create a space that felt tailor-made for my patients.

Over the course of several months, I scoured the antique shops of London for the finest furniture I could lay my hands on. Everything from the chairs to the carpets, the curtains and the tables came at a high price, and enabled me to create a waiting room dripping with a sense of exclusivity. I hired two assistants, both dressed in individually tailored outfits, who knew how to arrange flowers in a vase on the reception desk and make exquisite coffee for my clients. I even insisted that they grind the beans each time they made a fresh pot, so the aroma was as welcoming as my cushioned chairs. I bought the most expensive cups and saucers I could find, displayed potted plants in silver wine coolers and even applied the same level of care and attention to the ladies' restroom. I strongly believed that it was important to provide a private area for my female clientele that reinforced the sense that they had come to the very best practice in the city. To finish, just so everyone felt assured that they were in the hands of the very best dentist that Zurich could offer, I had my exam and postgraduate certificates photographed and transformed into sheets of wallpaper. Within this palace of oral hygiene, no patient was ever kept waiting. In fact, some were known to come without an appointment just to have the pleasure of sitting quietly in lovely surroundings and reading magazines that were never out of date.

Overall, my strategy had been heavily informed by my time in America. It was all about first impressions, and buying my clients' confidence, which allowed me to make savings when it came to purchasing dental equipment. I was very serious about my profession, and committed to earning a reputation that justified my scale of fees (controlled by the Swiss Dental Association). I just happened to have learned that expensive tools didn't buy good treatment. That was down to the skill of the practitioner, using simple, economical and trusted equipment, and remained my secret throughout a career that spanned almost forty years.

Over time, my client list came to boast film stars and artists, chairmen of the board, international investors and their families. There was no room for compromise and this was reflected in my growing status as a dentist to the rich and famous. My wife would assist me with the billing, and the figures she put together never failed to make me blink in disbelief. I worked incredibly hard to build my practice into a profitable business, and this was further fuelled by the additional responsibilities that arrived with the birth of our two sons, Christian and André. I was driven to provide, no matter what the cost.

Throughout my career, I crossed the Atlantic every year to attend dental conferences and seminars in America. In addition, I regularly visited the practices of the finest dentists in the US and watched how they worked. It was important to me that I should stay abreast of the very latest developments, techniques and debates. I also enjoyed the cultural differences, and very possibly a break from the routine of parenthood and work.

In the early years, I would attend a large meeting in Chicago. It was hosted in a hotel that boasted a splendid rank of elevators, and the girls who operated them always caught my eye. They were so fragrant, beautiful and magnificent to behold that I could miss my floor just admiring them. As the decades passed, and technology evolved, so the need for elevator operators became obsolete. With a control panel at your disposal, you just pushed the button for the floor you desired and travelled the lonely journey staring at your shoes. The lobby, however, was a different matter entirely. It was always packed with delegates. In order to marshal the flow of traffic, the hotel employed a squadron of terrifying women with scowls like a storm front to muscle us in and out of the next available elevator. They would snap, shove and shout, and it broke my heart.

'What happened to those sweet, adorable girls they used to employ here?' I asked a colleague on one occasion, as we straightened our ties having been manhandled into the elevator at ground level. 'How much has changed!'

My colleague smoothed his hair back into place and sighed. 'Nothing has changed,' he told me. 'They're the same girls. Just older.'

Time, it seemed, waited for nobody. I was just so focused on my work that I failed to pay proper attention to the effect it was having on me. Midway through my career, some time in the late 1960s, when I looked in the mirror I saw a man who could consider himself to be a success in his profession. I was financially secure, with a rewarding career and a shining family. That my hairline was receding from the shore of my brow and my waistline filling at the edges wasn't so much a sign of age. I saw it as a price worth paying for the lifestyle I provided my family.

Without realising, on the cusp of turning fifty, I had become a balding, self-satisfied lump of lard.

Now, there are some people who can blindly ignore such a mid-life transformation, and others who wake up one day and don't like what they see. I certainly reached that point, perhaps a little slowly and belatedly, and decided that something would have to be done. Although there was nothing I could do about my receding hairline, which served as a steady reminder that I wasn't getting any younger, I remained determined to get in shape.

With high hopes, I purchased a fitness manual designed for use by the Canadian Air Force (the *Royal Canadian Exercise 5BX Plan for Physical Fitness*, published in 1950 and later revised). It had been recommended to me as a practical handbook guaranteed to improve fitness without the use of any equipment. The book contained useful charts and diagrams, and presented workouts and exercises that were intense but effective. Unfortunately, in my enthusiasm I approached the task of toning my body in completely the wrong way. Quite simply, I failed to factor in any adequate recovery time between training sessions. I continued to push myself by following the book's instruction, until eventually something broke.

Tuberculosis is a highly infectious and life-threatening respiratory illness. Should you be fortunate enough to survive, it can compromise the immune system for a long time afterwards. Having overcome a bout during the war, I should have been more careful, but at that point I was caught up in a battle against middle age. The first indication that all was not well took the form of a cough. It was an irritation, but I couldn't afford to take time off work. Then my symptoms worsened, and I saw a doctor. When he made the diagnosis, having viewed an X-ray that showed a hole in my lung the size of an orange, I was given no choice when it came to the course of action available to me. In shock at this unwelcome relapse, I was packed off to a sanatorium in the Alps for a six-month period of rest and clean air. This time, however, I left behind a potential catastrophe in the making. Not only did my staff need to be informed so they could monitor their health, it was only right that the same warning should extend to every single patient on my list.

For six months, I felt as if my world was teetering on the verge of collapse. I'd left my family at home, and it was only thanks to some prudent insurance that I was able to retain my staff and appoint a young dentist to cover emergencies on my behalf. It was a deeply stressful time, which did nothing for my recovery. With the aid of a new antibiotic called Aureomycin, administered intravenously, my condition slowly improved. After a while, I was permitted short periods of free time. Most patients made the short walk down the mountain to the cafés in the village. Determined to hasten my departure, I went in the opposite direction by heading uphill.

I didn't venture far at first. I was too weak, and my time was limited. I also knew that if my doctors discovered what I was doing they would ground me immediately for the sake of my fragile health. But the longer I had available to me, and the stronger I felt, the further I dared to trek. Each time, I would plod up a winding track through the larches and pines, turn at an appropriate moment and run back down. This was my bid to get some air into my lungs and use my legs, and I found that I rather enjoyed it.

Every day I was allowed to leave the sanatorium, I

practised this routine religiously. Each time, I went a little further up the mountain. Eventually, I climbed as far as a mountaineer's hut overlooking the forest valleys and snow-capped ranges beyond. There, I rested for fifteen minutes, taking in the crisp, clear air, before embarking on a run through eight miles of trail back down to the sanatorium. It was an experience that proved to be both challenging and liberating. The trails were tough to negotiate and steep at times, but the connection with both nature and my body helped me to get back in touch with what was important in life. I felt it improved my lung function, but also the pure white and azure alpine vistas combined with the solitude and the rhythmic pace of my footfalls left me feeling cleansed and refreshed.

Just over six months after I was admitted, I left the sanatorium to pick up the pieces of my life at home and work. Back in the family fold, I fully expected to find my practice in ruins. Instead, much to my surprise, I found every single one of my patients had chosen to remain on my books. They considered the fact that I had notified them of my condition to be the mark of an honourable man, and for that I was both grateful and profoundly humbled. Having triggered a serious relapse in my health as a response to becoming middle-aged, I had returned as an enlightened man. I felt in good shape as a result of my mountain running, but now I appreciated just how important it was to allow time to recover in between exercising. How long depended on the type and intensity of the training, I learned, and this would become a source of fascination to me.

8

Late Summer

It's often said that we are at our most entrepreneurial in spirit between the ages of fifty-five and sixty-five. This age group is responsible for a significant number of startups across Europe and the USA, for example, and from experience I believe I know why.

Having run my own dental practice for over twenty-five years, I found myself drawn to exploring additional avenues in the field. I'd always enjoyed attending conferences and lectures in the USA, and I wanted to find a way to share the latest clinical findings, news, views and information. In the late 1970s, a clinical newsletter seemed the most effective way to communicate within the profession, and so at fifty-nine I set about putting one together in the evenings and weekends. To begin, I joined the American Newsletter Association and attended their meetings every year in Washington DC. I wrote and designed everything, established a small subscriber base, and then printed and posted a copy to each one. When that proved to be well received, bringing me a small return with potential for growth, I refined the format a little and even published it in French, as well as in German. I also rented a small office in Zurich that I used as a base for the work. Within a short space of time, what had started as a sideline interest became far bigger than I could have imagined.

And so, by accident as much as design, I found myself with a second job as I set out into my sixties that suited me just fine.

I was quite capable of balancing my commitments to the practice and the newsletter. My sons had grown up, and so I filled the space I would have otherwise devoted to being a father. It was hard work, but I had acquired sufficient experience, confidence and clarity of purpose to grow both businesses. Having stumbled as a response to reaching the middle of my life, I believe this is a virtue of that phase that we should not ignore.

Ironically, such a golden era of entrepreneurialism comes at a time when other aspects of our lives can begin to fall away.

In the ten years since my return to Zurich from the sanatorium, I had made every effort to look after my health. Having survived that second bout of tuberculosis, and supported my recovery through mountain trail runs, I maintained a sensible approach to keeping in shape. Instead of throwing myself full throttle into a quick-fix fitness programme, which had proved so catastrophically counterproductive, I felt that a return to a sport that had been so central to my early life might keep the effects of ageing at bay.

Aged sixty-three I found a rowing partner called Willy. Like me, he was in his early sixties, and on that basis we went out on the lake at Zurich and trained in a pair. It reminded me of my youth in lots of ways. I got up early in order to train before work, and came to appreciate sights and sounds at dawn that I would have otherwise missed. It made me feel better, from the moment I saw my first patient at half past eight in the morning to the time we closed for lunch. In Switzerland, we enjoyed a kind of alpine siesta that could last for two hours, and I made full use of this long lunchtime break in winter by returning to the lake. Without doubt, rowing helped me to feel good. Then I'd catch sight of my reflection and my spirits would sink. Eventually I had to concede that rowing was not going to furnish me with the body I desired. As an endurance sport, it placed demands on my aerobic capacity but did little in terms of helping me to shed the extra pounds.

From thirty onwards, it's estimated that we lose 3 to 5 per cent of muscle mass each decade. In effect, I had to work much harder than younger rowers to achieve a satisfactory performance. At the time, I regarded this not as an obstacle but a challenge. Throughout that period, however, my friend began to struggle. Although he rowed on a regular basis his performance fell away. I saw the same decline in another senior rowing acquaintance, Charlie D. While he tried in vain to improve, the physical deterioration was heartbreaking to witness. To make things even tougher for Willy, his mental faculties then slipped. In turn, when both men passed away, I looked at my life and worried I would be next. All I could think to do was keep pulling at those oars with all my might as if that might spare me the same fate. Such was my determination in fact that, as I headed into my seventies, I found more success in the sport than I ever had in the past.

The Masters Rowing Series permits entrants to compete by age category. For a long time, the focus had been on rowers in their prime, but at that time a range of age categories were introduced that catered for me. The opportunity was irresistible. I had been training to the best of my abilities over a long period. Six days a week, I would be out on the water whenever I could, working on my stroke and endurance capacity. At last here was a chance to see how I fared in competition once again! I had found someone prepared to row with me, and to our delight we were moderately successful in national regattas.

Through the years that followed, I participated in a number of international regattas. As time ticked by, I even found that I became more attractive as a rower. Unfortunately, this wasn't down to an outstanding ability but my advancing years. In Masters competition, teams are categorised by their average age. By including me in their boat, a team could afford to include younger rowers without dropping down into an arguably more competitive category. I thoroughly enjoyed being in demand, but for all my efforts I couldn't ignore the diminishing returns in my performance. By this time, some years after the loss of Willy and Charlie D, I knew exactly what was happening. Pulling the oars, it seemed, just wasn't going to save me.

While rowing is a test of endurance as much as skill, I had come to recognise that it doesn't build muscle. Despite their efforts in the boat, I had witnessed two elderly friends deteriorate with age. Now it seemed inevitable that I would follow suit. I even began to suspect that Willy's subsequent loss of mental capacity was linked somehow to muscle degeneration. Certainly my physical appearance was losing definition. My circulatory system was in great shape thanks to the demands placed on me by the sport, but I didn't look good. As a man with a long-standing habit of appraising himself in the mirror, it meant I also didn't feel good about myself. It was as if age had let me down, at a time when I was busy and professionally fulfilled with my dental practice and newsletter. Quite simply, I didn't want to just give up! As it turned out, however, this unflinching dedication to my work was set to contribute to another significant change in my life.

With great sadness, having raised two fantastic sons together and after many years of marriage, Edda Bianca and I decided to separate.

Early in the 1990s, it became clear that we could no longer be together. It was a traumatic time in many different ways. Financially and emotionally, it left me stripped to the bone. Looking back, my feelings about that episode are very different now compared to then. Today, by contrast, I feel nothing but gratitude towards my ex-wife. Despite the circumstances in which we parted company, it heralded a new direction for me that I wouldn't change for the world. With great fondness and sincerity, I am happy the experience proved just as liberating for Edda Bianca. We all change over time. Our needs and values evolve, and sometimes that makes us incompatible with people central to our lives. But that doesn't mean we must lose sight of the good times we shared, or allow the new opportunities we afford ourselves to be overshadowed. It's a question of taking responsibility for our feelings, no matter how painful that might be.

In the aftermath of my divorce, in my early seventies, I found myself living in a small, sparsely furnished flat in Zurich. It was the kind of place I might have been comfortable in as a younger man. At the time it seemed so wretched. I had few belongings to my name, and feelings that would take some time to process. Crucially – and this was my lifeline – I still possessed the means to earn an income. Following our divorce, I redoubled my efforts at the dental practice. Working with a spirited new chair-side assistant whose punky hair was no reflection of her work ethic, I managed to double my gross income. As well as making money, my aim was to become a better dentist. I valued my patients for their loyalty, not least when I had fallen ill, and I went on to become friends with many of them.

One of my clients was a famous German novelist. He was such a fabulous raconteur that I would often book him in for a double appointment simply so I could listen to his stories. On learning of my personal situation, he offered advice that I took to heart so I wouldn't make the same mistakes again.

'There are just three words that will save a relationship,' he told me. 'You. Are. Right.'

Every evening, when the practice closed, I would head back to the flat. Instead of winding down at the end of a busy day, however, I focused on producing the next newsletter. Often, this would take me until eleven or twelve at night. I was growing my readership with every issue, and ploughing the profits back into the business in order to make it more sustainable. In a way, it felt like raising a third child. At the time, it certainly felt as rewarding.

My commitment to work might have played a part in the end of my marriage, but afterwards it enabled me to get back on my feet. At an age when my peers were winding down, I spent more time with patients at the practice and at my desk in the flat than ever before, and loved every minute of it. By rights, I could have retired in my mid-sixties. It simply hadn't occurred to me at the time, and then the divorce meant work was a necessity once again. It wasn't just financially rewarding, however. In terms of my mental wellbeing, my roles as a dentist and with the newsletter presented me with challenges, goals and a sense of satisfaction that I was struggling to find on the water.

I freely admit that I was lonely during this time. Having spent so much of my life in a marriage, I found it difficult to settle with being single. Happily, just two years after my divorce, I met the love of my later life.

Elsie was an anglophile. She loved everything about the country and the culture, which rather put me at an advantage. At her request, I would read her *Alice in Wonderland* and a dreamlike expression always crossed her face. She was a beauty and a most wonderful human being. At her invitation, I moved into her house in the hills just outside Zurich to begin a wonderful time in my life. I was still working hard at the practice, but I didn't want that to come between us. So I asked Elsie if she would assist me as my secretary. To my delight, she agreed! Not only that, she shone in the role. After feeling so derailed in the wake of my divorce, I felt as if I had found my soul mate. In due course, we were married and I could not have been happier.

On reaching seventy-five, I finally turned my attention to the prospect of retirement. My dexterity was beginning to be an issue when working with precision dental instruments. With the quality of my work in mind, I knew it was time to stop. Having paid into the pension pot throughout my life, I did at least feel prepared in some ways, and so I made the decision to close the doors for the final time. It was a bittersweet moment, but I still had the newsletter. More importantly, Elsie and I had plans. With so much free time available to us, I looked upon my life after dentistry like a late summer had just arrived.

We were very happy together in the years that followed, though I wasn't so keen on my reflection in the mirror. It was as if closing my practice had been a cue for my body to seemingly deteriorate before my eyes. Nevertheless, my relationship was in fine shape. Elsie was a sociable soul. She could light up a room with conversation and always sought positive qualities in everything. She had a longstanding girlfriend from school, and they spent a great deal of time together. On one occasion, they decided to go on a driving holiday to France. While Elsie was excited by the prospect, I worried about their safety. The fact was her friend was a terrible driver. When I raised this with Elsie, she offered to drive. This did little for my confidence, because Elsie wasn't much better behind the wheel. I even presented her with an article about the high number of deaths on French roads. Elsie brushed away my concerns. They would be fine, she assured me, and continued to pack ahead of their journey. Once I'd seen them off, I headed back inside wondering how I might fill the short time while she was away. Without her, the apartment felt very lonely.

At some point in the days that followed, my dear wife and her friend were involved in a collision with a lorry at a junction in France. They were both killed instantly. I was eighty-two when I lost Elsie. It felt like I had died with her.

9

Game Over

As a widower, whenever I looked into the future I could not see beyond a handful of bleak and final years. Alone in the house, and conscious that my body was seriously failing me, I became convinced that I would die at eighty-five. I had little to live for, it seemed, and duly began to wind down in preparation.

Soon after my wife passed away, I published and distributed my final newsletter at eighty-two. I no longer had the heart to continue with it. What was once a burning passion just seemed like a chore. It meant little to me any more. When I reflect on that period it's quite clear to me now that I was depressed. In grief, however, it's hard to see things with such clarity.

Life is simply dominated by what is no longer there.

Throughout this time, as if clinging to a semblance of my life before loss, I continued to visit the lake six days a week and take part in World Masters rowing events. Competing in the 80-plus category, I couldn't ignore the fact that the competition had thinned considerably. Sometimes I would enter an event and be assured of a medal position before I'd even dipped my oars in the water. My performance, however, continued to disappoint me. Despite my commitment to training, I felt I was failing to fire on all cylinders. My muscles were wasting away and slowly turning to fat. I was putting on weight for the wrong reasons, all of which contributed to feeling plain wretched. It seemed I was as washed up on water as I had become on dry land, and that was hard to accept. At the time, rowing was all I had.

In a moment of reflection, I decided that perhaps I could build on that by finding work at a local sports club. It was an idea that unexpectedly filled me with a sense of hope. It had been a long time since I felt that way as I knocked on the secretary's door and waited for her to summon me in.

'I was wondering whether you had any job vacancies,' I said.

She looked me up and down as if seeking some indication that I might be joking.

'Like what?' she asked after a moment.

'I'll consider anything,' I told her.

The secretary held my gaze for a moment longer, which effectively left me to find my own answer. There I was, a man in his mid-eighties who was willing and able to work. The way I felt just then, I might as well have been volunteering for a trip to Mars. In terms of my outlook on life as much as my prospects of finding employment, it was game over.

With no work to keep me busy, I had plenty of opportunity to think and dwell on my situation. It began to dawn on me that my experience of retirement was in stark contrast to my expectations. Losing my wife had not been part of the plan, of course, but the lack of work coupled with my diminishing physical abilities combined to leave me feeling thoroughly adrift. I had nothing to anchor me, no purpose or goal. I even failed to die at eighty-five! The year just came and went, and I filled it by living up to type as a cantankerous old man. I might have closed my practice and my newsletter, but I remained a member of various dental associations. As a result, I would receive everything from magazines to AGM minutes, and took issue with any rule, regulation or point of contention that I could find. I became a prolific writer of letters driven by pedantry and point-scoring. Why? The answer was very simple, and I knew it then as I do now: I simply wanted something to do.

Throughout my life, I had never been unemployed until this moment. Now, in my eighties, supposedly enjoying the gentle pleasure of retirement, I felt as if I had opted into an illusion. I was bored and inactive, and both served to accelerate the decline in my physical function. Every winter I would pick up a cold, and each time I would take longer to shake it off. Financially, I was relying on my health insurance for medical care and living off annuities, though I was in no doubt that people like me who were unlucky enough not to expire placed a strain on the providers. I was, in effect, a bet that had failed to pay off for the insurance companies who targeted me, and just one of a growing number of old-timers that were undermining the foundations of that business model.

Pacing the house, I would think about my situation in a wider context. Surely I wasn't alone in finding that later life had become a struggle for the reasons that were supposed to enhance it? To fill my time, I began to read papers on issues central to my concerns, from the economic unsustainability of the pension industry to the physical and mental consequences of inactivity in old age. As a life Fellow of the Royal Society of Medicine, I arranged for a steady stream of research abstracts to be sent to me from all over the world on the subject of ageing, as well as sport and exercise, and nutritional supplements for muscle building in the elderly.

Increasingly, what I found opened my eyes to a situation that we cannot allow to continue. Not only was it apparent to me that the medical profession has limited insight into training and exercise for the older generation, I began to pull my ideas together and distil them into one fundamental conviction. Quite simply, our concept of retirement is little more than a slow death sentence.

For the sake of future generations, I realised, we have to transform what it means to be old.

Ironically, pensioned retirement is a relatively youthful proposition. It only took shape in the mid-nineteenth century, when public and private programmes were introduced across American industries. By paying into a scheme throughout their lives, workers could look forward to security in their final years while ensuring a healthy turnover in the labour market. Beforehand, people were expected to stay in their jobs until they had enough money to retire, or died, and so this attractive alternative quickly became a fixture in our life cycles.

Europe soon caught on to the model. In Germany, a retirement age of seventy was first introduced at the turn of the twentieth century when average life expectancy was forty-six. Under strange and almost comical circumstances, this was reduced to sixty-five in 1916 in that country, following widespread misinterpretation of a comment by a leading scientist of the day. During a speech in Oxford, one Professor Olser in 1910 referred to a dystopian novel by Anthony Trollope called *The Fixed Period* in which the male inhabitants of an island community were regarded as useless on reaching sixty and subsequently euthanised. While Osler made the reference in a moment of light-heartedness, the press seized upon it and reported that men were worthless at sixty-four. Fortunately, the government didn't take such drastic measures, but in due course the age at which citizens were dispatched from the workforce duly came down in line with a vision effectively set out in a work of fiction. From here on out, the concept of being paid to wind down in later life began to seep into the public consciousness. Just after the Second World War, however, retirement went viral.

With millions of soldiers demobbed, demand for jobs outstripped availability. In response, the government sought to encourage the older generation to hang up their work boots with the promise of a pension, thereby making room at the entry end of the labour market. As the average life expectancy was also sixty-five at the time, it made the system entirely sustainable. You worked hard, enjoyed a couple of years of supported living if you were one of the fortunate to exceed your expected time in the world, and that was it.

Then, thanks to advances in medicine, industry and society, we started living longer, and the countdown to our current disaster in waiting began.

In the years between 1965 and 2005, life expectancy in forty-three selected countries rose by an average of nine years. During this period the average retirement age across these countries increased by only six months. So, for the retirement model to remain fit for purpose, we all need to work harder before booking that cruise.

Sadly, this just hasn't happened. Today the maximum working week is forty-eight hours, with an addition of 20+ days of paid holiday and various national or religious holidays each year. Can this amount of work be expected to fund a retirement lasting 25–30 years? Of course not, and the consequences are devastating. Not only will that fleeting cruise fail to keep you occupied for the rest of your projected life, the present pension schemes are financially unsustainable for both the private sector and the state. It is absurd that we should spend about a third of our lives being unproductive and supported by other people's children. The enormous growth in the numbers of the aged, coupled with the rapid expansion in the global population, makes the present pension system unaffordable.

Despite this, we are still wedded to the concept that our later lives will effectively be paid leisure time.

There is, of course, an argument that we're not fit for work beyond sixty-five. Health and socio-economic factors may play a role in some cases, but it's by no means a rule with any scientific basis behind it. For many, reaching that age has no bearing on fitness, health or productivity, and yet an aspect of modern life that has proven so fulfilling must come to an abrupt end. It's as if we reach an expiry date, determined by government, with no individual assessment. One day you're in an office, maybe as a manager running a business, and the next you're surplus to requirements. As well as the financial implications, should you go on to live for decades, how does this make you feel? Such a sudden loss of usefulness and self-esteem can have a profound impact, and we're rarely prepared to deal with it. In my opinion, what's needed isn't a carriage clock or a bunch of flowers but a period of counselling to help people come to terms with what they're facing.

In addition, drawing on a pension makes it almost impossible for you to increase your income. This is dangerous. You have put yourself in a precarious situation. Even if you can find employment or be self-employed, you will be faced, in most countries, with deductions from your state pension or additional taxes. Quite simply, you have chosen dependency instead of independence.

Then there is the question of whether your pension pot is going to be big enough. In the US, for example, the funding gap for all state pension schemes is estimated at $4 trillion or 25 per cent of GDP. This is a terrifying gulf. The estimated return on pension fund assets is assumed to be 7.5 per cent, yet Treasury bonds, for example, only yield 2 per cent. With some pensions at risk of being chronically underfunded, only a huge increase in taxation will plug the gap, and yet when politicians are presented with the facts they simply sweep the problem under the carpet. Pension liabilities are not even to be found on the balance sheet.

In looking into the reality of retirement, I found myself feeling cheated. The idea of what might be regarded as a long-term funded holiday seemed so wonderful, especially having worked into my mid-seventies as a dentist and until eighty-two as a publisher. This is reinforced by a sense that we deserve it after having invested so much in our careers. Perhaps the greatest selling point is that it enables us to spend more time with our families (but why should they be punished?), on hobbies and travel, while state and private pensions pick up the bill. On paper, it is undoubtedly an attractive prospect, but the grim reality is that our increased lifespan has undermined the system. Setting aside any setbacks in our personal lives, it traps us in a wilderness with only one way out.

In my opinion, society has failed to adapt to an ageing population. It has made a complete mess of the fact that we will live longer than we have ever done before. Twenty per cent of those living today are expected to reach 100, and in the vast majority of cases we are still quite fit and able to work beyond sixty-five. I might have experienced dexterity challenges in my seventies, but looking back there was no call for me to close my practice altogether. It was simply the done thing before I finally eased into retirement. Only then did I open my eyes to the reality of the situation. I might even have continued with my newsletter had I not been in a dark place following Elsie's death. Once I'd come to terms with my loss, however, and attempted to rejoin the workplace, it became quite clear to me that any attempt was futile. I was too old, in the eyes of society, which I regard as an injustice to this day. Instead of making an active contribution to my world, I had nothing to look forward to but a feeling that I had outlived any useful purpose.

My experience is not unique. Man has destroyed the joy and wonder of ageing by transforming it into a time of relentless degeneration and disease. Today, the aged are overweight, over-medicated and physically and mentally inactive. How did this happen?

Our bodies are still close to those of the Palaeolithic era when we were hunter-gatherers. Food was so scarce that as much food as possible was consumed. The excess was stored as fat, but only so that would enable us to survive the next famine. As humans at this time faced such physical and mental demands, unnecessary activity was avoided. Today, with an excess of food, and with survival no longer dependent on huge physical and mental effort, our instincts still tell us to consume an excess of food and avoid activity as much as possible. Those instincts that in the past enabled us to survive are now destroying us.

While my winter colds became progressively harder to overcome, I found evidence to suggest it was wrong to assume that any illness at this time of life is simply a product of old age. The fact is *inactivity* is the culprit, just as it was for my weight gain, after I gave up my newsletter. To understand this, we must recognise that work, health and wellbeing are closely and powerfully linked. Statistics show that employment, particularly in seniors, is associated with a low disease burden, while the unemployed visit a doctor more frequently. Why? Because the loss of structured daily activity that generally comes with retirement also means a drop in occupational energy expenditure – and this is fundamental to a healthy life. It should therefore come as no surprise to learn that on giving up their careers the retired are at an increased risk of suffering from chronic disease and depression. In my view, retirement is little more than an incubator for illness and health problems. It's a social experiment, I think, that has led to unintended and negative consequences. By extension, work can be therapeutic. For young or old, it can reverse the adverse health effects associated with unemployment.

We have misused retirement, I believe. It's unaffordable, creates invalids on a massive scale and could devastate our present health systems. Retirement also denies society the potential and expertise of pensioners. Ultimately, it's a destructive waste of talent. As a social experiment with good intentions, it has now gone horribly wrong with devastating social, economic and personal consequences. The fact is retirement has been linked to a future 20 per cent reduction in the standard of living. If we are to continue insisting that at sixty-five we cease to be productive, and must rely on state and private funding, then we need a rise in taxation and contributions to fund it that will be frankly unacceptable to the electorate. Without it, however, we can only expect an increase in national public debt, the risk of negative credit ratings as a country and potential caps on medical costs. Coupled with the damage to your personal health, not only due to being unemployed but to a lack of mental and physical activity, there is simply no benefit to anyone in retirement in its current guise.

The good news is that an alternative approach exists that benefits both the individual and wider society. Having found myself at rock bottom after everything fell apart, something stopped me from simply giving up altogether. Driven partly by a sense of outrage at my situation, and my longstanding vanity that proved so troubling every time I faced a mirror, I took steps to change my life. Duly, I picked myself up, shone a light into my future and trod a path I believe that anyone can follow if they're willing. To my great surprise, and infinite relief, I found the experience to be productive, sustainable and rewarding on every level.

I may not have known it as I set out to reinvent myself, but my best years were ahead of me.

Part Two

Second Life

10

A New Beginning

Curiously, I first began to feel more positive as the truth about retirement dawned on me. It took some time to reach my conclusions, but the process proved invigorating.

I wanted to change things, and not just on a personal level. I knew for sure that I wasn't alone in feeling as if my age somehow excluded me from fulfilling my potential. For far too long, we have looked upon the elderly as a generation that offers nothing but requires constant support, and this seemed quite wrong to me. I offered very little as a member of society through much of my eighties, but in passing the year I expected to die a strange kind of rebirth occurred. Reflecting on the pension crisis, and the health issues associated with retirement, I started to think constructively. The idea that we should all stop working and put our feet up had to be replaced with a vision that enabled the elderly to play to their strengths and fulfil their true potential. Gradually, I found myself focused on three areas that I believed would come together to support an outcome I call 'successful ageing'. Let's discuss them in turn.

Work

Each year, about 650,000 people turn sixty-five and walk away from the workplace. In addition, over twelve million people are of state pension age (currently sixty-five for men and rising for women from sixty-two to the same age by 2018), which is almost one in five of the UK's total population. This means there are more pensioners than children under sixteen, and that number will continue to grow.

In the next twenty-five years the number of people aged sixty or over in the UK is projected to rise by over 50 per cent. By 2031, it could pass the 20 million mark. That's a lot of old-timers.

It would be easy to interpret these figures as proof that our quality of life is improving. We're growing older than ever before, after all! But my concern is what we're doing with this bonus time, and the impact it's having on our society. The future economic strength of a country is determined by, amongst other things, the percentage of the population considered to be productive. It means those countries with a projected increase in the number of aged are therefore deemed to have a poor future prognosis. The elderly are considered not only to be unproductive but an enormous burden on health services. My response is very simple. Enable this redundant generation to return to work.

We know that unemployment causes chronic disease and mental problems, as well as poor health, disability, more medical consultations, more medication and more hospital admissions. While the aged are often regarded as vulnerable, any issues they're likely to suffer are seriously compounded by retirement. The beneficial physical demands that accompany any job are removed, from travel time to shuttling between meetings, for example. As a result, the pensioner is rendered inactive in every way.

In any role and industry, work is therapeutic. It might not seem that way at times, but there are wide-ranging benefits that often go unappreciated. Not only is it an intrinsic part of improving and maintaining physical health, as well as stimulating mental and social skills, it's a determinant of self-worth, family esteem, identity, and standing in the community.

In theory, it's hard to argue with the economics of returning the elderly to the workplace. In reality, the proposition inevitably meets resistance from several quarters. An increase in retirement age and a reduced pension is politically difficult. In practice, however, it could be made more attractive by offering retraining or new opportunities to post-retirees in order to help them re-engage with work in a realistic, meaningful and rewarding way. At the same time, we must flag up the wider benefits of work so it doesn't become the grind that often happens when we lose sight of our objectives. Without doubt, the increase in activity, financial and emotional reward can only increase your chances of feeling fulfilled through later life. It's a question of repositioning the concept of work in an attractive light – and there are undoubtedly benefits – and then helping and supporting the older generation to feel valued and connected on every level.

While the blessings of a working retirement have been underestimated, I believe the horror of being elderly and idle has been completely overlooked. It's an existence defined by loss, from social status to the satisfaction of earning money and the prospect of slow mental and physical decline. If we look at the figures associated with dementia, for example, in which the number of cases doubles every five years from retirement age, then effectively we have a time bomb on our hands. In the 65–74 age group, chronic disease becomes an issue we can't ignore. The cost to our society is enormous, with over three-quarters of all health spending devoted to treating the elderly.

As we shall see, the discovery of the enormous plasticity of the human body means that it is possible to rebuild one's body and mental powers in old age through specific exercises and changes in diet. This in turn will not only prevent decline but can increase physical and mental powers. Thus the possibility of work in old age together with fewer demands on the health services could be feasible.

Furthermore, the aged are an increasing political force. In the US the numbers of voters over the age of sixty-five represent 17 per cent of the voting population, but as they vote more regularly, their share of the electorate is already 20 per cent. In the next two decades this will rise to 30 per cent. Politicians as much as influencers who seek innovative ways to meet the needs of the elderly could well find themselves at an advantage.

Your old age can be an incredible opportunity, and not simply a period of degeneration before an inevitable end. I believe that in years to come you can be an asset instead of a liability. Talent development, together with the future work environment, will enable you to work far longer than has been thought possible until now. In many ways, this isn't the end but a new beginning.

You also have a head start over the younger generation, in that the 55–65 age group are often regarded as the most entrepreneurial. I count myself as having contributed to this figure. On starting my newsletter, at a time when others think about slowing down, I called upon decades of experience, wisdom and confidence to turn a sideline into a profitable business. Chances are this is something I just wouldn't have been placed to achieve as a younger man. In many ways, the time as much as the confidence to see a project through is something that comes with age. While there may be little difference in the early growth performance of startups between younger and older founders, more of the enterprises established by the latter group are still in existence after five years.

Of course, entrepreneurialism isn't for everyone. I am also well aware that many people can't think of anything worse than staying in their hated job for another couple of decades. My response is to view what we consider to be the age of retirement as an opportunity to assess where you've come from and plot where you're heading. In many ways, we're making the most important decisions of our lives here. Maybe this is a time to retrain, or try a new line of work that builds upon your skills, talents and creativity and expands them as you take on new challenges. Everyone is different, of course. Some people are constantly hungry to take on new responsibilities, while others might be only too happy to downgrade to a post or position that simply allows them to feel valued and active.

In order to achieve this, we need a climate in which the elderly are celebrated for their wisdom, experience and demonstrable commitment to work. This will require measured debate and a dialogue between all governments and the people they govern, because ultimately we, as taxpayers, employees and employers, foot the bill.

It won't be an easy task to convince you that everyone will have to work longer, retire later and give up more of their earnings to provide for themselves in later life. But we need to change our attitude towards retirement and old age so that it is no longer seen as the justification to put your feet up and rely on state-provided benefits. It should be the time when your new talents can be developed, coupled with continuous learning. Learning prevents the shortening of your telomeres (the caps at the end of each strand of DNA that protect our chromosomes). Shorter telomeres have a negative effect on our health. Learning benefits your health. In addition, it should also be the moment we take more responsibility for our health.

Nutrition

I'd like to begin by distinguishing between nutrition and diet. When we talk about the food we eat we're concerning ourselves with diet. Nutrition focuses on what's in that food, and the impact it can have on our health. Both are equally important, of course, but I believe we should be looking at nutrients as the critical component of successful ageing. In my view, antioxidants like vitamins C, E, and the pro-vitamin A (beta-carotene) play a vital role, as do folic acid, vitamins B6 and B12, zinc, calcium and vitamin D. These are all available naturally with a sensible eating plan. Unfortunately, we're living in an age where our attitudes to food and nutritional content have caused an unprecedented global health crisis.

As human beings, we are citizens of the Palaeolithic era when humans were hunter-gatherers. Today, in the twenty-first century, those who better match with an active lifestyle will likely have a longer life expectancy and a reduced risk of chronic disease. However, the daily activity energy expenditure of most individuals in contemporary western societies is only around 38 per cent that of our ancestors. While it's a fact that strenuous endurance exercise improves life expectancy, we're simply not doing enough. Today our lifestyle has created energy imbalances that undoubtedly contribute to chronic disease. At the same time, environmental pollution has increased drastically, which means our produce is compromised nutritionally. Although our forefathers had heavy expenditures of energy, their food was rich in vitamins and minerals, but not as dense in calories as modern food. As well as requiring some effort to hunt or gather, it was also less plentiful. So it's no coincidence, I believe, that we were in better shape back then. But that doesn't mean we should just accept poor diets as an unfortunate product of the age, particularly at a time of life when good nutrition is so vital to health and welfare.

It's very easy, as we all know, to fall into bad habits. We might turn to processed food or ready meals for the sake of convenience, but in doing so we're playing fast and loose with fat and excess calories. It's estimated that 50 per cent of US Americans and Canadians are either overweight or obese. Should trends continue then 100 per cent will be either overweight or obese by 2048, and the rest of the western world isn't far behind.

We have a big problem with weight in the western world. Our waistlines are expanding, through a combination of factors such as poor diet and exercise, and this is effectively killing us. Nowhere is this more apparent than in later life, when weight-related issues can cause health complications and impact on our quality of life.

Chances are if you consider yourself to be overweight then you're worried about your waistline. In reality, the real wake-up call takes the form of visceral fat, and this can often be an invisible threat to our health. Visceral fat invades inner organs such as the liver, pancreas, intestines, heart and kidneys. Even muscles can be streaked with fat, just like your bacon rasher for breakfast. Obviously, if the organs concerned have been invaded by fat then they cannot function properly. In addition, visceral fat produces toxins. For example a substance called interleukin-6 doesn't just disrupt the normal balance and functioning of hormones, it also causes chronic systemic inflammation. This condition in old age is termed 'inflammaging' and is related to a deterioration of the immune system. Together with the malfunctioning of the inner organs this can give rise to chronic disease. It's a prospect which should give us all pause for thought, and that extends to the biggest killer of them all.

Obesity caused by a poor diet – along with a sedentary lifestyle – is one of the main causes of type 2 diabetes. Complications often prove fatal, such as a heart attack or stroke. In addition, there is a risk of blindness, kidney failure and even amputations. There is even some research that suggests that in obesity the prefrontal part of the brain shrinks! Most frightening of all, however, is just how widespread the problem has become.

At present, we have a global diabetic pandemic affecting 8.5 per cent of the world's population. It's worth noting that many experts believe that only half of the cases worldwide have been diagnosed. They also agree that the number is escalating rapidly. In the USA, diabetes is now diagnosed at a rate 90 per cent higher than a decade ago, with associated healthcare costs doubling over the same time period. What's more, the western diet and lifestyle is fast being adopted by developing countries such as China, India and Indonesia. The result is that already 10 per cent of the population of China alone (or 134 million people) are diabetic. In short, we are eating ourselves into a life of disease, and placing huge burdens on the healthcare system.

The cost of diabetes treatment runs into billions in both Europe and America. It already stands at 11.6 per cent of world healthcare, which is frankly unsustainable. If you think that your health insurance will cover treatment costs then you are probably mistaken. The fact is our present healthcare systems will soon be unaffordable. In the future, you may well have to pay for at least part of your treatment. The next time you opt for a cheap and cheerful burger, consider the fact that an illness related to your diet could ruin you financially.

The good news for the overweight is that it's possible to lose both the subcutaneous and the visceral fat with the aid of diet and exercise. Not only do you increase your chances of saving yourself from chronic disease, you will have made a contribution in the fight against the diabetes pandemic.

Without a shadow of a doubt, the food you eat can have a huge impact on the quality of your later life. As muscle mass begins to fall away with age, for example, it's important to eat food rich in protein, such as fish, eggs and (in my opinion) meat. In conjunction with a specified exercise regime, this will help rebuild lost muscle, and yet older people tend to consume a diet rich in carbohydrate like potatoes and bread.

Of course, the key to all diets is balance. That means a mix of food rich in carbohydrate *and* protein, and not too sweet, not too much, not too salty and not too fatty! Ultimately, when it comes to good nutrition the best expert to help tailor a diet specific to your health and wellbeing is your doctor. They can help you to build and review a sensible eating plan that puts your health and welfare first, and may also recommend a nutritionist to work with you. Consider it the fuel, if you like, in your bid to age successfully.

Exercise

As I have learned from experience, vanity is a much-maligned character attribute. There have been several stages in my life when I didn't like the way I looked, as indeed there would be once again as I neared my nineties. In seeking to improve my appearance through appropriate exercise, I found that I took care of my health as a welcome bonus. The rewards are holistic, and I would encourage you to consider the benefits with regard to ageing successfully.

We know that loss of muscle mass occurs with age. Known as sarcopenia, it's one of the most debilitating factors of later life, and has even been classified as a disease. The natural response to sarcopenia is to get fit, but as I saw in my friends Willy and Charlie D, aerobic exercise such as rowing is ineffective. What's required is a means of *rebuilding* muscle, and this can be achieved through hypertrophy-specific exercise. What we're talking about here is intense, regular strength or resistance workouts that promote muscle growth. It's a regenerative process. Muscles are also known to release messenger substances to the brain and ultimately promote growth hormones. From personal experience, when combined with protein and animo-acid supplements, I have found this approach has had a profound, life-enhancing effect with widespread benefits. Let's examine them in turn.

- **Longevity**: According to a twenty-year study, regular exercise reduces the risk of dying prematurely. In short, if you are physically active then chances are you will live longer.

- **Disease prevention**: Exercise can be a major factor in the prevention of disease. Although it should be stressed that factors such as genetics can impact on individual responses, research has shown that it can reduce the risk of certain conditions including heart disease, stroke, colon cancer, type 2 diabetes and hypertension significantly.

- **Help for chronic disease**: The list of conditions which can show improvement, or whose symptoms may be improved with regular, carefully targeted exercise continues to grow. While it should be stated that 20 per cent of the aged are classed as 'non-responders' to strength or hypertrophy exercises, the 'responders' may well find it goes beyond physical improvements. As well as combating sarcopenia, exercise can be beneficial to individuals with heart disease, chronic obstructive pulmonary disease (COPD), lung disease, breast cancer, bowel cancer, cerebrovascular disease, diabetes, rheumatoid arthritis, osteoarthritis and osteoporosis.

- **New brain cell development, improved cognition and memory**: It's a fact that exercise stimulates the formation of new brain cells, while learning something new can have significant neurological benefits (and it's never too late to take on a new challenge!). Researchers have found that the areas of the brain that are stimulated through exercise are responsible for memory and learning. For instance, older adults who engage in regular physical activity have better performances in tests involving decision-making processes, memory and problem solving. In short, exercise can improve not just your body but your brain by boosting white matter.

- **Improved sexual function and better sex life**: If you take regular exercise it may maintain or even improve your sex life. Physical improvements in muscle strength and tone, endurance, body composition and cardiovascular function can all enhance sexual functioning in both men and women. Researchers have revealed that men who exercise regularly are less likely to have erectile dysfunction and impotence. Resistance and hypertrophy exercises are also associated with testosterone increase.

- **Exercise is a powerful antidepressant**: Study after study has shown that exercise promotes mental health and reduces symptoms of depression. Just be aware that it may take at least thirty minutes of exercise a day for at least three to five days a week to significantly improve symptoms of depression. But then if you want to improve your life and your old age you'll be planning on doing at least this amount of exercise every week, if not more!

- **Cardiovascular health**: Lack of physical activity is one of the major risk factors for cardiovascular diseases. Regular exercising makes your heart, like any other muscle, stronger, and endurance exercise is particularly effective here. A stronger heart can pump more blood with less effort.

- **Cholesterol lowering effect**: Exercise itself does not burn off your cholesterol like it does with fat. However, it does improve blood cholesterol levels by decreasing LDL (bad) cholesterol, triglycerides and total cholesterol and increasing HDL (good) cholesterol. A combination of aerobic and resistance exercises and diet control is recommended.

- **Prevention and control of diabetes**: There is strong evidence that moderate physical activity combined with weight loss and balanced diet can potentially cause a 50–60 per cent reduction in the risk of developing diabetes. The expected improvement in glycaemic control with exercise has not been clearly demonstrated, but aerobic and resistance exercise have been shown in many cases to help reduce the risk of or control diabetes respectively.

- **Blood pressure lowering**: The ways in which exercise reduces blood pressure are unclear, but regular exercise can be beneficial. Aerobic exercise appears to have a slightly greater effect on blood pressure in hypertensive individuals. But unfortunately there is evidence suggesting that exercise can worsen the condition in some people – another very good reason to take medical advice before undertaking any form of exercise.

- **Reduced risk of stroke**: Research data indicates that moderate and high levels of physical activity may reduce your risk of total, ischemic, and haemorrhagic strokes. For example one study indicates that highly active individuals have a 27 per cent less incidence of stroke.

- **Weight control**: Regular exercise can help you to reach and maintain a healthy weight. If you take in more calories than needed in a day, exercise offsets a caloric overload and controls body weight. It speeds the rate of energy use, resulting in increased metabolism. When metabolism increases through exercise, you will maintain the faster rate for longer periods of a day. Ultimately, exercise combined with diet control is the best way to reduce weight.

- **Bone strength**: Your active lifestyle benefits bone density. Regular weight-bearing exercise promotes bone formation, delays bone loss and may protect against osteoporosis – the form of bone loss associated with ageing. Unfortunately exercise has been a disappointment in preventing osteoporosis in women.

- **A better night's sleep**: If you suffer from poor sleep, daily exercise can make the difference. The natural dip in body temperature five to six hours after exercise may help you to fall asleep.

Exercise is both a preventive measure and a treatment. It's also, I find, a great enabler. I'm particularly drawn to research showing that those who participate in strenuous competitive sports live longer. Not only is training more intense, which can greatly enhance successful ageing, the competitive environment gives rise to valuable adrenalin rushes, coping skills, teamwork, friendship, confidence and a great sense of achievement. I find my increasing age has only driven me to broaden my horizons by taking on new sports and pursuits. If I can do it, so can you.

Ultimately, exercise can be very successful not only in increasing health and fitness in the old but also for disease treatment and prevention. With work, diet and exercise, I believe your body can be completely rebuilt at any age.

And on turning eighty-seven, having emerged from a desolate phase of my life feeling wiser and enlightened, I set about doing exactly that.

11

More Body!

Just one thing kept me anchored in the years following Elsie's death, and that was rowing. While I spent a great deal of time in solitude, either reflecting on the perils of retirement or making a nuisance of myself writing abrasive letters to dental associations, I continued to go out on the water regularly.

The decline in my performance proved steady and depressing, but I didn't give up. In many ways, rowing was a lifeline. It provided me with the chance to be sociable, and feel needed as part of a crew. In my sixties and seventies, I had been an attractive proposition as a competition oarsman because my age could bump a team into an older category. On reaching my eighties, I proved irresistible! No doubt I made little contribution, but my presence on the boat was seen as being advantageous to a crew several years younger than me. We were all veterans, of course, but their ability to pull an oar left me painfully aware of my shortcomings.

It also left me determined to do something about it.

In all my research into ageing, and the potential pathway to making it a rewarding experience, I was particularly drawn to studies of the physical deterioration of the human body in terms of both cause and effect. I knew for a fact that from the age of fifty we begin to lose muscle and increase fat. That certainly felt like my experience as I struggled to perform on the water. I was rowing nearly six days a week, and yet I no longer possessed the capacity to pull the oar satisfactorily. Unwilling to simply accept the situation, I was extremely interested to learn that all was not lost. And so, at eighty-seven, I set out to lose the flab and acquire the kind of muscle many people my age assume to be an impossible task.

I just knew that I couldn't do it alone.

'You wish to do what?'

The man I had come to see asked me to repeat myself. It was quite hard to be heard clearly amid the sound of clanking and grunting as human specimens all around me heaved and pumped at weights.

'I want a beach body,' I told him. 'There are beautiful seventy-year-old girls out there, and I'd like to turn their heads.'

The figure looking down at me said nothing for a moment. Shaven-headed, with a neck and torso that looked to be bound tight under the skin by steel ropes, he folded his great arms and considered me.

'A beach body,' he said, as if to check he had heard me correctly. 'How old are you, sir?'

I saw no reason to be economical with the truth.

'Will you help me?' I added, in no mood to waste time. At my age, I just didn't have that luxury.

I had come to a gym in Zurich to see François Gay. As a bodybuilder, he had climbed to the pinnacle of his career on being crowned Mr Universe. In my bid to transform my physical appearance, it seemed only sensible that I should start at the top with someone who knew exactly what that entailed. The man was quite literally triangular, with clinically blue eyes that appraised my sagging, weathered frame.

'Get undressed,' he said after a moment.

If his question served as a test, I wasn't going to fail at this early stage. Folding my glasses away, I duly stripped down to my underwear and then stood as if awaiting a military inspection. I was well aware that I had very little to offer, but focused straight ahead as he looked over my miserable body. Finally, François began to nod to himself.

'It won't be easy,' he told me. 'Are you quite sure you know what you're letting yourself in for?'

'Whatever it takes,' I said. 'I have no job to keep me busy, so I'm all yours.'

He smiled, just for a fleeting moment, and then laid out his terms and conditions. He would establish a programme for me, so he said, on condition that I followed his advice to the letter. It would be intense, he promised. No doubt I would hate him at times, but if I wanted a body that turned heads on the beach those were the terms. I agreed without hesitation, thanked him for taking me on, and left wondering what on earth I had done.

I was prepared for the physical challenge. Having grown so fed up with my failing body, I knew that I would be required to push myself to the limit in order to achieve the desired results. In order to burn fat and restore muscle, I was well aware that I would have to put in more effort than most on account of my age. This was no quick-fix solution that might work for someone in their prime, and that was all part of the deal. What troubled me was François's demand that as part of his programme I would be expected to rest two to three times each week. As a rower, dependent on endurance fitness, I had spent decades training six days a week. Now, I was being asked to take time off between gym sessions and do absolutely nothing. I recognised that when it came to strength training this was the recovery period in which muscle would be built, but it didn't sit comfortably with me. Nevertheless, I was determined to honour my promise to François, and prove to him that I was a project that could achieve results.

My first task, following instructions from my muscle-bound mentor, was to lose weight. As fat would be the first thing to go, burned off through a combination of intense workouts and a change to my diet, I embraced the challenge wholeheartedly. In terms of eating, François advised me to cut out absolutely everything fatty, salty or sweet and simply reduce the amount on my plate at mealtimes. I did exactly as I was told, while attending the gym three times a week. The exercises he prescribed for me consisted of continuous resistance strength exercises using the machines at my disposal. Undertaking eight to ten repetitions each time, I focused on everything from my biceps to my deltoids, triceps, glutes, hamstrings and calves. Following Mr Gay's instructions, which he presented to me as a written programme, I worked on each muscle set to the point of exhaustion before moving onto the next repetition on his list. I greatly restricted my diet.

As a result of my efforts, every month I would climb on the scales to learn that I had lost a kilogram in weight. This continued every month for a year. By the end of that period, having shed 12 kilos, I was beginning to see noticeable results. I looked better, and felt much improved in my mind. François even suggested that I was close to being 'stage worthy'. Frankly that prospect frightened me, and I was content with feeling good. This sense of wellbeing should not be underestimated. It's associated with the stimulation of various hormones by physical activity, some of which occur naturally during adolescence. In America, and at enormous expense, injections based on testosterone are made available by doctors promising to rejuvenate older patients, and yet here I was getting my own anti-ageing hit for free! As a bonus, and this came as a complete surprise, my libido returned with a passion. Incredibly, I even found the grey hairs around my crown jewels regained their colour! What had felt like a guttering candle flame began to burn brightly once again, and yet even this wasn't enough. Despite everything, I still didn't possess a body that would cause those indescribably attractive young seventy-somethings to drop their jaws in amazement. There was just one course of action available to me. I would have to work much harder.

Throughout the following year, I spent so much

time in the gym rather than out in the clear alpine sunshine that I developed a vitamin D deficiency. This was easily resolved by taking a supplement, but it wasn't the only one I added to my diet. François was adamant that if I wanted muscle growth then I needed additional protein in order to build it. In old age, he explained, protein synthesis is reduced and supplements are necessary, including certain amino acids such as leucine. Placing myself entirely in his care, I did as I was told and began taking supplements in the form of whey powder mixed into a protein shake. While I might have been sceptical at first, the resulting improvement in my physical form demonstrated just how important it was to get the balance of my diet exactly right. Where I'd once carried fat I now boasted muscle, but rather than feel that I had completed my mission it simply left me more determined to make the most of my time in the gym.

By now, François had invited me to build free weight training into my regime, in order to improve my coordination and balance, which I embraced with gusto. I did so at my own risk, following careful instruction, and within a short space of time considered myself to be quite at home pumping iron.

You would be forgiven for thinking that I stood out as an oddity in this environment. There I was in my late eighties with pecs I could twitch and flex, and yet I was accepted into the fold. While many bodybuilders had to balance working out with demands from work or family, I was at least free to commit myself to the time my physical transformation required. The gym, in effect, became my office.

I continued to row, of course, despite cutting back on the time spent on the water. My fellow oarsmen admired the change in my physique, and I certainly felt a confidence boost as I pulled through the water. Nevertheless, I couldn't ignore the fact that my performance simply didn't come up to the exacting targets I had set myself. For all the effort I put into working out, and the sacrifices I had made regarding my diet, it seemed to me that I could still do better. I sported muscles that could be easily identified from the labels on the machines that had helped to create them, but somehow as a whole they didn't come together as I had imagined. It reminded me of the conversation I'd had back in America many decades earlier, on trading in my beloved Chevrolet for the Oldsmobile that would accompany me back to Europe.

'What do I get for my money?' I had asked the salesman on the forecourt, for the trade-in would require me to hand over two thousand dollars above the value of my Chevy.

The salesman had regarded me like the answer was staring me in the face. He rested his hand on top of the Oldsmobile and beamed at me.

'More car,' he said.

I had never forgotten his disarmingly simple response, and it echoed in my thoughts as I considered how far I'd come from the clapped-out codger who had showed up at the gym. After spending the best part of two years cycling through the machines and weight routines, I began to wonder whether this was really a means to an end, or perhaps a stepping stone on a greater quest. I had built an enviable body in terms of form, but what I sought for my rowing was function.

I had the physique but lacked the performance power. I needed more body.

I pondered this for some time. Then, on tearing a muscle that forced me to rest completely, I formed a plan of action. Throughout my time under François's tutelage, I had kept a close record of my activities that he reviewed once a week. In between, I effectively worked out on my own. My injury had come about through nobody else's fault. I had pushed myself too hard without sufficiently preparing myself for the task in hand. In a sense, it felt like I had inflated a balloon too far. If I was to achieve the outcome I really desired, one that went beyond anything I could sculpt in a gym, then what I needed was a performance expert at my side when I climbed back on my horse. François had done a fabulous job as a bodybuilding mentor, and continues to enjoy a stellar career with clients such as Paris Hilton. He had set me on the path to reinventing myself in a way that I had never dreamed would be possible. But now it was time for me to take things even further, which is when a formidable woman came into my life and promptly turned it upside down.

12

A Race of my Own

'Your bottom, Charles, is a *catastrophe*!'

I turned to face my critic. After years of bodybuilding, I didn't think my backside was that bad, but my new personal trainer clearly thought otherwise.

'Can you save it?' I asked.

I was eighty-nine years old, and about to be taken under the wing of a blonde, tracksuited former national gymnast from Austria nearly thirty years my junior. From that moment until the present day, Sylvia Gattiker has never told me anything is impossible, and so we set to work.

It was Sylvia who contacted me. She called one day after I had made some enquiries about a championship contest testing strength and flexibility. Having worked so hard in the gym, I was keen to see how I might shape up in competition. This particular contest had appealed to me greatly, especially because entrants were divided into age categories. When I rang to see if I could take part, however, and informed them I was about to turn ninety, it seemed to me that their enthusiasm dimmed by a degree. Somehow, Sylvia heard about my interest and took it upon herself to get in touch. Whether she was struck by my bodybuilding background, my continued attempt to rekindle my rowing performance, or simply wanted to help out an elderly man with a disastrous derriere, I will never know. From my perspective, however, I was impressed by her unique combination of experience in the field of sport and personal fitness, along with her master's degree in prevention and health management. In rebuilding my body in later life, Sylvia offered me an academic enquiry into ageing and fitness that also embraced the practicalities with great vigour, and I never once looked back.

So, rather than rely on machines to plump and tone particular muscles, we focused on hypertrophy-specific training to increase muscle size while exercising them in *groups*. With Sylvia at my side, counting me through everything from squats to crunches, chin-ups, pull-ups, push-ups, planks, thrusts and lunges, I worked through a programme designed to improve not just body shape but coordination and performance. In her view, controlled muscle and strength exercises formed the foundation for good health and physical ability. Functional training, as she called it, was the key to making the most of life.

During this time, I learned that even one simple exercise can be done in so many ways to give completely different results. A simple biceps curl, for example, with palms up holding a dumbbell and repeated a large number of times, can improve endurance. Increasing the resistance gives strength, while fast concentric movement (such as a biceps curl with a dumbbell) and slow eccentric movement (bringing the dumbbell back down) give coordination. Then there's slow eccentric movement to exhaustion, which often forms the basis of hypertrophy-specific training exercises. I discovered that the strength of muscle can be increased without increasing mass. But with increased mass comes increased strength. Together with Sylvia, I found myself in a whole new world of learning and relished every moment.

Saropenia results in a loss of power, strength and muscle mass. Loss of power can be compensated with plyometric exercises (exerting maximum force in a short period of time) and the loss of strength and muscle

141

mass can be compensated with hypertrophy training. In the bodybuilding gym, my muscles had been trained once to exhaustion. With Sylvia we experimented. One method was called 'the pyramid'. This involved training to exhaustion, repeating with less resistance to exhaustion and then repeating again with even less resistance to exhaustion. Another method demanded that I should train to exhaustion, wait sixty seconds and then repeat with the same resistance. In combination with protein supplements and amino acids, I found the second method gave me better results. Within months, turning to appraise my backside in the mirror, I began to consider myself almost ready for the beach. But not only did I look good, in my opinion, I felt stronger and by turns better than ever.

Alongside my training routine, and with Sylvia's help, I even managed to take part in the strength and flexibility competition that first brought us together. Qualifying in the 90-plus category, I had just one rival. While he didn't provide much competition, I greatly respected his participation. I just wished there could have been more of us. It had been nearly five years since I set out to reinvent myself. I was making great progress, and continually refining my diet to fuel my endeavours. My only regret was that I had not started earlier. If I could do it, I thought, as I took on the first of the competition's challenges that day, so could anyone from my generation. There was no question in my mind that it had been easy getting this far. Those five years had required dedication and effort, but ultimately I felt years younger than my peers.

The competition tested each entrant across a range of exercises, all of which I had practised as part of my regular routine with Sylvia. While I had to undertake the same exercises as competitors in younger categories, with the same number of potential points available for performance, some concessions were made for my age. When it came to the push-ups, for example, I was permitted to perform these with my knees on the ground. Likewise, I was allowed to keep my feet on the ground when I grasped the bar to do chin-ups, while the weights I had to lift were lighter than those presented to my younger competitors. While it was perhaps a sensible precaution, it certainly made things easier for me. Not only did I come top of my age category, I amassed a haul of points that placed me in contention to be the overall winner!

Having called the organisers on a whim, I left that competition feeling victorious for several reasons. It would prove to be an annual event for me, and since that debut year I have even won the championship.

On the water, I continued to apply demanding

standards to myself. Even as I turned ninety, I remained determined to pull my weight as an oarsman. My seniority still drew me into crews keen to tip their average age into a higher category, but now I felt as if I could make a useful contribution once again. In that time I amassed over thirty Masters gold medals in races across Europe and as far afield as Canada. I am in no doubt that my commitment to redefining my body was responsible for such an achievement. Had I not focused my training on improving muscle mass, my performance wouldn't just have carried on declining with age. I am convinced I would have simply withered and died.

Nevertheless, as I reached my mid-nineties, the demands placed on me in competitive rowing began to take a toll. Back problems became an issue for me, perhaps inevitably after years of pursuing an endurance sport, but it was my heart that sounded a serious warning sign. This took the form of an irregular heartbeat and feelings of breathlessness during a race in Poland. It left me feeling quite unwell and also mindful of my age. Sylvia had shown me how important it was to push myself within a sensible, informed framework, and her approach had brought me fantastic results. I was duly careful in my recovery, and even felt much better on my return to competitive rowing. But when I ran into the same trouble once more, almost a year later during a race in Italy, I realised that perhaps it was finally time to lay down my oars for good.

I once had a great friend who shared my passion for rowing. Like me, he had continued in old age. Residing in Paris, where he remained an active club member, he went out alone on the Seine on one occasion. I could just imagine him cutting through the water, cocooned in his own blissful world, passing under bridges, with a unique view of the capital's great buildings. He was never seen alive again. Four days later, his body was recovered from the water, having suffered a cardiac arrest. While I have no doubt he died doing something that he loved, his passing left a deep impression upon me. Unwilling to risk following in his wake, I donated my sculling boat to the rowing club.

Walking away from the water's edge was bittersweet. I had achieved a great deal in a sport that defined my life until this moment. It had shaped my youth, tided me over through middle age and then returned as a pillar of my later years. I was desperate to find some kind of workaround that would keep me in a boat, but couldn't avoid the reality of the situation. Due to age, my body was no longer cut out for the repetitive endurance demands of my beloved pursuit.

No doubt on that day many people assumed I would

shuffle off into the sunset and reflect on my former glories. Without question, it was a painful and sad moment in my life, but I had amassed enough experience over the years to know that for every door that closes another cracks open and a bright light shines through.

By now, Sylvia had come to consider me as a long-term experiment into training regimes for older athletes. As I'd been delivering results, and relished the pioneering journey we'd undertaken together, she had no intention of letting me go despite this setback. She was also sensitive to how much rowing had meant to me, and so we sat down to review my situation. While I was in great physical shape, the endurance demands of the sport were too great for a man of my vintage. I possessed the muscle to pull the oars, but doing so over a sustained period was no longer appropriate. I read up on the subject hungrily. I accepted that endurance sport was a step too far for me now. It was no longer appropriate for me to power through the water for long periods of time. On learning that cardio patients in recovery benefited from very short bursts of high intensity training, however, I knew I was on to something straight away.

'Running?' said Sylvia when I shared my findings.

'*Sprinting*,' I said to be more specific. 'Fast and furious!' Sprinting training is high intensity interval training.

My reasoning was based on the classic physique

of the distance runner. This was someone who was characteristically lean in build and carried as little weight as possible. By contrast, the great sprinters were constructed like powerhouses: muscular, with broad shoulders and limbs primed to propel them forward with explosive intensity. Having learned from experience that muscle mass in old age is effectively an elixir, I knew precisely where I wished to devote my attention. Under supervision from Sylvia, who was well aware that the World Health Organisation recommends only moderate intensity training for the elderly, I believed I had discovered another way to showcase the virtues of successful ageing. Sprinting would be a completely new experience for me, a rarity for a man in his mid-nineties, but I relished the challenge to showcase high intensity interval training for the elderly.

As time was of the essence – as it had been since I defied death at eighty-five – I decided to start at the top. Despite never having run in competition in my life, I took steps to enter a championship meeting at national level.

The British Masters Athletics Federation is the governing body overseeing official events in the UK. Even as I made the call, enquiring as to how I might submit my application, I was ready for them to express surprise at my age. Increasingly, this had become a source of frustration for me. Just because I was very old, I failed to see why I should not be considered an athlete in the same light as someone in their prime.

'So that would put you in the 95-plus category,' the person on the other end of the line told me, before falling silent for a moment. 'We don't have anyone in that category you can run against. I'm afraid the rules won't allow you to compete in a race on your own.'

This didn't seem like an insurmountable objection to me, and indeed my friend on the phone quickly came round to my way of thinking.

'Could I run alongside another category?' I asked.

'Well ... we could put you in a lane with the 70-plus.'

'That sounds fine.'

'Seventy-plus women.'

'Perfect!' I declared, before ending our call.

Even though I'd yet to earn myself the body that would turn heads on the beach, those septuagenarians of my dreams would surely notice me on the track.

I am often asked what preparation I undertook ahead of my debut in the world of championship sprinting. The honest answer is very little. The nearest track to me in Switzerland was so far away it wasn't realistic to train there. So mostly I spent the time in planning and paperwork. Having secured my place, I booked tickets for Sylvia and me to fly to the UK ahead of the meeting, and we just showed up on the day.

Of course, I had done plenty of research beforehand. Not only would I be alone in representing the 95-plus category, I learned that nobody in this group had ever actually covered such a distance at a championship in the UK. Quietly, as I took my position for the 100-metre outdoor event, I realised that meant if I could just cross the finishing line alive then I would become a game-changer.

I don't remember much from when the gun went off for that first race in my sprinting career. I just recall being caught up in a whirlwind of veteran female runners, all of whom left me for dust. It was certainly a test of my male pride. I'm not even sure they noticed my presence on the track, let alone my body! Then again, I wasn't competing in the same race as them. So I just got my head down and pushed on to the best of my abilities.

I crossed the finish line 25.76 seconds later, with a British record for my age. Not that taking the title was on my mind at the time. The sheer exertion left me exhausted. It was only when people rushed to congratulate me that I realised what I had achieved. Usain Bolt, Linford Christie, Carl Lewis and every other 100-metre champion now had a new name in their ranks. To think that person was me left me beaming with pride. It might have taken me an extra fifteen seconds or so to get over the line, but when it came to these legends I was old enough to be their grandfather.

Unfortunately, that moment of glory didn't last long.

'The rules state that you must be a member of a British club for the record to stand,' said the official.

'I belong to a club,' I told him hotly. 'Thames Rowing Club!'

'It has to be an athletics club,' he said in a tone that I can only describe as apologetically bureaucratic.

I know when to pick my fights, and this was not the moment. While the record didn't stand I had still become British champion for my age category. Later that day, I went on to claim the same title in the 200 metres with a time of 58.03. Sylvia was waiting for me at the finish line, and once I'd got my breath back we celebrated just how far we'd come. My place in the record books would have to wait, however, and I knew that deep down I would not rest until I had a chance to give it my best shot.

13

Beyond the Finish Line

Ten years had passed since I woke up to the horror of retirement. In that time, I had gone from a low point of feeling redundant, out of shape and effectively waiting to die, to a fit and motivated 95-year-old with an ever-expanding trophy cabinet. I had reinvented my body and fundamentally changed my diet. I wasn't on some restrictive regime that offered me no pleasure. I just ate according to my needs, enjoying every meal, and felt rejuvenated as a result.

What's more, as I became more vocal in my belief that successful ageing was within everybody's reach, I even received an offer of employment at the age of ninety! This was an important moment for me.

I considered myself to be able and willing to work, as indeed do many people who take retirement and then realise they have sacrificed something intrinsic to their life. Naturally, I accepted the invitation without hesitation.

In a sense, it was my sporting achievements that served to bring me to the attention of an employer. With every win, on the water and in tests of strength and flexibility, I built a reputation as one of the world's fittest pensioners. Increasingly, I was invited to talk about the subject to a range of audiences, and relished every chance that came my way. As is often the case, one thing led to another and I was approached to become a public face for one of the largest European chains of gymnasiums. The company were keen to promote muscle building for all age groups, including the elderly. In many ways, it was regarded as a groundbreaking outlook, and one I was enrolled to support by giving lectures and attending trade shows. Delighted to be in employment once again, I even found a new use for the little office in Zurich I had used as a base for my newsletter. Rather than spend all my time in the house, I would set out on foot up the hill, catch a train, then another train and then a tram into the city, and put in a day's work at my desk researching the ageing process. Even after my contract came to an end after two years, I found the regular commute and sense of purpose contributed to my wellbeing, and so I continued to make full use of it in attending to correspondence and paperwork. In my view, a place usually abandoned at retirement had become a vital lifeline for me.

When I wasn't at home or in the office, I devoted my efforts to working out under Sylvia's guidance, and then training for my next sprint challenge. This time, before entering the British Masters Championship at Lee Valley on the outskirts of north-east London, I took the precaution of joining a recognised athletics club. I wasn't upset or bitter at missing out on the British record back in Birmingham. For me, the most important thing was that I had thoroughly enjoyed the experience. On what would be my next attempt, however, if I stood a chance of going faster than anyone else in my age category had gone before, then I didn't want to find the finish line crossed with red tape. And so I joined an organisation whose name helped me feel like I belonged: the Veterans Athletic Club of London.

Several months before Sylvia and I travelled to the UK for my second British Masters championship, I began to focus on improving my sprint performance. While we worked on the muscle groups that would help to power me, I wanted to put in time on a track. With no such resource within easy reach, I took matters into my own hands and created my own.

I live on a steep, winding hill on the fringes of mountainous forests. It's beautiful up there; peaceful and clean, an opportunity to find solitude in nature. So, whenever I had the chance, I laced up my trail running shoes and plodded up towards the fringe of trees. There, I explored several winding tracks until I found a long, narrow glade. By my reckoning, it was sufficient for me to pick up a decent speed. So, quite alone but content in my surroundings, I set about practising. I'd count myself off from a makeshift start line and then hurl myself through slanted beams of sunshine to reach the other end. There, I'd catch my breath before repeating the process. Back and forth I'd go until exhaustion set in. Then I'd trudge home and make a pot of green tea. This was my routine several times throughout each week come rain, shine or snow. Sometimes the ground underfoot was muddy. On other occasions, it was hard packed or even frozen. With nobody to watch me but the wildlife, I ran every attempt with one goal in mind: to perform to the best of my abilities when it mattered most.

It never occurred to me that I should change my trail running shoes ahead of the race. They were certainly becoming worn, but still felt comfortable on the uneven forest floor. As I had run in nothing else, I just packed them in my bag without further thought. It was only when we arrived at Lee Valley, an indoor stadium sporting a banked track, that I began to wonder if I was properly equipped. Ahead of the race, my two fellow competitors had joined me to walk a lap. I noticed these old boys had brought running spikes with them, which they left at the start line along with their power drinks. It was the first time I had ever seen such a fancy pair of shoes. Until that moment, I didn't even know spikes existed.

Having traded the tranquillity of the forest for the stadium, and the constant hum of chatter from the spectators, I told myself not to worry about my shoes and just concentrate on what I had to do. Even with ninety-six years behind me, and countless competitions, I still had nerves to manage. So I reminded myself that the two athletes with their spikes were in a younger category than me, and not running the same race. I was in competition with myself as much as with the traditional view that the very old were fit for nothing but a comfortable seat in the sunny spot at the care home. If I could change the opinion of just one person in this stadium, I thought to myself, it would all be worthwhile.

'Good luck,' said Sylvia, when I had completed my exploratory circuit.

By then, I was in the zone. Having laced up my shoes, and made sure my spectacles were tight around my ears, I was ready to assemble at the start line.

'See you on the other side,' I said as she set me off with a pat on my back.

From that moment on, in front of a crowd in a covered and cavernous stadium, I felt just as alone as I did in the glade, and for that reason quite prepared. I had come a long way to be here. Whatever the outcome, it would be the race of my life.

The opening half lap disappeared in a blur. Coming under starter's orders seemed like a distant memory, as did the first hundred metres and the banking that delivered me here – to this moment where I began my story – on the back straight with a seemingly impossible task ahead of me.

'Come on, Charles! Run!'

So this is where you find me. My legs have turned to lead weights. My chest heaves with every breath I haul into my lungs, and yet it doesn't feel like enough. All I can do is call upon the growing vocal support from the crowd and convert it into energy.

I swear at the start I heard nothing from the spectators. Maybe I was just so locked on to the challenge ahead that I failed to register their presence at all. Now I can't ignore the rising wave of cheers, whoops and whistles that carry my name. It's as if perhaps they've only just noticed the elderly back marker running his heart out, despite the fact that the other two veteran athletes on track are in the closing seconds of their race.

'Go, Charles! You can do it!'

I lift my chin, determined not to give up now despite every fibre in my body urging me to do so. By now I've reached the second bank, only this time I know what to expect and simply push with all my might. The track levels off once more, unlike my sense that I'm on the limit, and suddenly there it is. Ahead of me, a white line across the track that marks the point at which this torment I'm putting myself through can finally come to an end. My vision is tunnelling, but I can distinctly make out my two competitors on the other side of that line. They're at a standstill, hands on hips as they reclaim their breath, which is all I want to do.

'Run, Charles!'

The sound of my breathing and final footfalls are entirely drowned out by the din. I know I'm fading but nothing will stop me now, and when I hurl myself across that line it takes a moment for me to realise I have finished. I slow to a walk, annoyed with myself because I believe I could have trained harder for that final push, and then stop to rest my hands on my knees. I am exhausted. My knees feel no stronger than butter curls. Despite my frustration, I know for a fact that I have nothing left in reserve. Every drop of energy that I possessed went into circling that track as fast as I could. I might have set out like a gazelle in my mind, but I'm resigned to the fact that I must have looked like some awful shuffling old man. Now all I have to do is get my breath back and hope I don't keel over in front of all these people.

'Well done, sir. That's quite a result.'

One of my fellow competitors has approached me. I look up, shake his hand and offer him my congratulations. The other fellow is close behind. He looks as exhausted as me, but on pumping my hand he draws my attention to the timing board. In focusing on the finish line and nothing more, I had completely forgotten about my time. I squint through my spectacles as he walks away. As I wait for the LED digits to stop swimming before my eyes, I hear Sylvia calling for my attention. I turn to see her jumping up and down with excitement.

'You did it, Charles! 55.48 seconds! That's a world record!'

My trainer's excitement takes a moment for me to

translate. When it dawns on me what I've just done, I simply find myself grinning from ear to ear.

'Well, that's nice,' I say, as Sylvia rushes across the track towards me.

'So, how does it feel?' she asks when I finally extract myself from her embrace. 'Now you're a world champion?'

By now, the applause from the crowd has subsided. A long jump event is taking place inside the track, and attention has already turned to the next competitor. It comes as a relief to feel like I'm out of the spotlight. I might have just made history in my own small way, and I'll continue to break records on the track from that day forth. Just then, however, after everything I put into taking this first title, not just physically but mentally, there's only one thing I want to do.

'I might just go back to my hotel room,' I tell Sylvia.

'To celebrate?' she asks.

'For a nap!' I declare, as if a man of my age could wish for anything more at the end of such a glorious day.

Part Three

Your Life

14

A Long, Hard Look in the Mirror

Health and fitness in old age is unfortunately a great rarity. Even so, it does exist in a few odd places such as Abkhasia (South Caucasus), Vilcabamba (Ecuador), Hunza (Pakistan) and Okinawa (Japan). The people of these regions are mostly farmers in difficult terrain. They have a job. They have endurance and even hypertrophy exercise. They have natural food. They are not retired. Such examples from very different parts of the world show that an excellent quality of life in our later years is achievable. That it's regarded as unusual in the western world is an indictment of our lifestyle, health, social services and the medical profession.

It is generally accepted that old age is accompanied by inevitable disability and serious illness. In my view, chronic disease is not related to age but to retirement – and I hope I have demonstrated that I am living proof.

It is a fact that strength, coordination, balance and even muscle mass can be dramatically increased in the aged in a very short time by exercise. Not only is exercise an excellent means of maintaining good health. I believe it can also have a role in the treatment of chronic disease. Although there is a great deal of evidence to support this, inactivity among the aged has been allowed to become the fourth highest cause of preventable mortality. In the same way, our diet in later life becomes more critical than ever before. In old age, protein synthesis is reduced and yet modifications have not been implemented or propagated. Instead, we are overloaded with carbohydrates and this has severe health consequences.

In my bid to kick against the expectation of what later life should be like, I have found that sometimes even the medical profession isn't equipped to support efforts to age successfully. On turning ninety, while training under Sylvia's watchful eye, I undertook a health test to be sure everything was functioning as it should be. A doctor in a check-up centre discovered that my haemoglobin levels were low, and immediately assumed that such an elderly patient must have been suffering from anaemia. He advised me to take iron supplements, but these had no effect. As a consequence, I was sent to Zurich by the head haematologist to be checked out at a specialist clinic. There, it was finally established that my blood is thinner simply because it needs to flow quicker. The condition is termed 'Sports Anaemia' or 'Dilutional Anaemia' and is common with athletes. In the same way, rowers or weightlifters often experience 'Exertional Haemolysis' whereby the older blood cells are removed to increase the number of young cells. Once the doctor was wise to the facts, his concern turned to praise and admiration at my efforts, but I found the experience to be extremely revealing. The blunt truth is that doctors are just not familiar with the idea that the very old have the capacity to take it upon themselves to become fit and healthy.

Now, if I can achieve results like this in later life, then you have every opportunity to do the same thing and more. It's just a shame that you might be ahead of the medical profession in proving that the elderly have as much potential to improve their lives through exercise and nutrition as anyone else. No doubt they will catch up as more of us show what can be done, and the benefits that can be gained not only on an individual level but for the wider society.

Which brings me back to work.

While exercise and diet are critical to successful ageing, it is a fact that unemployment is associated with health issues such as chronic disease and mental problems. On the other hand, research has shown that work and health are intertwined, and yet at a certain age we're encouraged to drop one of these vital pillars of our existence. Upon retirement one's job, occupation or profession is often forcefully removed. There is little or no opportunity to develop dormant talents, learn a new profession or to find gainful employment after retirement age. It's not only detrimental to health and a financial disaster, I feel it's a shocking waste of talent and human potential. Fortunately, I was able to find employment at ninety, become a speaker at ninety-three and an author at ninety-seven.

Ultimately, not enough is being done to promote active and working lifestyles in old age. The main problem is the fact that too little is known. Research on physical activity, diet or even the effect of work on health is practically non-existent above the age of seventy. While responsibility rests with research facilities and promotion by government as well as health agencies, it's a shocking fact that there are far too few healthy individuals above the age of eighty to be able to conduct meaningful research.

For now, I'd like to take the lead by sharing advice and suggestions for successful ageing based on my experience. I would like to think it will inspire you to do a little bit more exercise and encourage others around you to do the same. Let's get you up on your feet, active and a valued member of society rather than the drain that everyone else sees us as.

So, this is the moment where we turn our attention from my adventures in successful ageing to an action plan for you. Together with my trainer, Sylvia, I have devised a guide to the trinity of components that form the foundation for a later life lived to the full: *work*, *nutrition* and *exercise*.

Naturally, as human beings we are each unique. There is no one-size-fits-all solution, but what I can offer you is a springboard of practical information and advice to help you launch a strategy tailor-made for you. For some, this might mean minor adjustments to an already active existence. Others might take a long, hard look in the mirror and recognise that they need to make a significant transformation.

In making any change to your life, the first thing to register is that only you are capable of achieving it. Nobody can force you to do this. I just hope that reading about my experience might encourage you to reflect on your experience and ask if there's room for improvement.

Often this begins by recognising where you are now. Whether you're looking at retirement or you've crossed that threshold, such self-searching might well give rise to uncomfortable truths. This can only be a good thing. It means you're more likely to be inspired to make positive changes.

In every case, whatever changes you're considering, it's vital that you put your health first. This means you should always consult your doctor beforehand and then check in with them on a regular basis. Even if you're just thinking about taking on work once again, you owe it to yourself to make sure it's appropriate. Ultimately, in terms of optimising your health and welfare, you should consider your GP to be part of your team.

So, in encouraging you to devise a programme for successful ageing, I'd like to begin by grasping an uncomfortable truth. Statistically only 5 per cent of the UK population meet the minimum physical activity recommendations. This means that if you consider yourself to be an average person then chances are your diet and exercise habits need overhauling. In effect, your lifestyle could be shortening the number of years you have left. What's more – and if you're seeking motivation to make a change then this could be what persuades you to act now – it might well be casting the same shadow over your children and your children's children.

Mothers and fathers of overweight and obese children are often found to be heavier than the parents of normal weight children. Parents and the lives they lead have a huge influence on their children. At the same time, grandparents can also be role models.

So, does it matter if your grandkids are fat? It does. Eighty per cent of overweight children aged 10–15 are obese by the time they turn 25. It seems clear that one of the main causes is the poor lifestyle of the adults in their lives as they grow up.

Your grandchildren's health and lives are under threat. This is a fact we have to recognise, but not accept. We can help to improve things for the next generation. Essentially, if you change your lifestyle then you are not only giving yourself a new life but your actions could influence the health of future generations. Frankly, the way you live your life influences the lives of others and our future. And when you realise you can live your life more healthily you will often find that you don't have to do very much to achieve it. In effect, it's a question of being more mindful of exercise and diet, and then finding a job if possible. That's all there is to it!

As a catalyst for change, it's worth establishing

several goals. Alongside a desire to safeguard the health of future generations, you might well find motivation from reasons that are individual to you. Do you want to show your children that you can fit into those smart clothes you last wore ten years ago? Would you like to be able to go on a long walk with your grandchildren, and not feel like you're holding them back? These are simple objectives, but with the right approach they're entirely achievable.

The point is that you can change your body. It can be modified, refined and improved. Not only will you look better, and feel better about yourself, it can help you to kick-start a whole new chapter in your life. Ultimately, it could encourage you to develop interests, skills and talents that until this moment were simply a dream.

Age is just a number

Let's begin our assessment by recognising where we are in life, specifically in terms of age. While we're not getting any younger, it shouldn't be a source of embarrassment. We're simply talking about the number of years we've been on this earth, and though time passes at the same rate for us all, there's often a big difference between the number of candles on a birthday cake and how we actually feel.

Often, the age of possible retirement is when you're categorised as being a 'senior citizen'. In some instances, people choose to stop work earlier, but does that make them over the hill and all washed up? The answer is not just in the mind but in your physical state of health. In every case, building muscle mass is essential for your physical welfare, and getting fit is the path to feeling good.

In establishing a guide that aims to help you identify how you shape up according to your years, let's start at a turning point in life. It might mark the age of early retirement for some, and this could be anything from fifty-five upwards, but if my experience has helped to enlighten you then it can become a moment of rebirth.

55–64: The early years

Having lived for over half a century, perhaps raised a family and seen them grow up, you've arrived at a stage where you can pause for breath. You might feel like you've come a long way, but in reality if you're prepared to seize every opportunity then the best is yet to come. In terms of physical welfare, it's worth noting that the loss of muscle mass, also known as sarcopenia, begins around thirty and continues at a rate of between 3 and 5 per cent each decade. At the age of sixty, you can expect to have lost 15 per cent of your muscle mass. By recognising this now, and taking steps to rebuild lost muscle, you'll be setting yourself up for a quality of life that might have been denied to you had you decided it was time to shift down a gear. It's often said that an old car needs a good drive to clear carbon build-up from the engine. In my view, the same approach applies to humans.

It's also worth reminding ourselves that this is the age group that boasts the fastest rising number of self-employed workers and the highest rate of entre-preneurial activity. In the USA, it's estimated that there are twice the number of tech startup founders aged fifty and over compared to those aged twenty-five and under. Clearly, experience and opportunity work in favour of the older generation here, but these facts also speak volumes about drive and determination. So don't compare yourself to younger, often louder models and write yourself off. You have a great deal to offer, and this could be your time to shine.

Not only are these early years a golden opportunity for starting a new venture, statistics show that they're also likely to endure. Seventy per cent of the companies founded by the 55–64 age group last more than five years, compared to only 28 per cent of those founded by younger generations. From personal experience, when I launched my newsletter at the age of fifty-nine I felt better placed to do so than at any other time in my life. I could call upon an established career as a dentist (which had taught me to understand and value my customers) and possessed the confidence to give it my best shot. In doing so, I grew the venture into a profitable, long-standing business. My only regret is that I chose to pack it in at a low moment in my eighties. I sold the business, in fact, and it collapsed soon afterwards. Sometimes, your DNA is so invested within the soul of an enterprise that it cannot survive in anyone else's hands. I have no doubt that had I stuck with the newsletter through that difficult personal time, it would have carried me through and enabled me to work until the present day on something that brought me rewards beyond simple monetary gain. Starting a new venture is like giving birth, I think. It will grow like a child and take on a life of its own, which is amazing to experience.

At about sixty some very important decisions have to be made. Chances are this is why you're reading this book. It concerns your future for potentially thirty years or even more. The decisions you take will decide whether future ageing will be successful or not. If you recognise that retirement can be a devastating experience then you need to take steps now. This means thinking about whether the work you're in at this present time will sustain you through the years to come, or whether this should be an opportunity to retrain for a different position or occupation. Should you find that despite everything the prospect of retiring is too good to resist (and in my opinion it's largely a financially unsustainable fantasy), then you must find a way to compensate for the drop in a measurement known as energy expenditure.

The World Health Organisation (WHO) recommends a minimum weekly activity expenditure for all adults. This doesn't just cover work but home and leisure time, but clearly if you're in some form of employment then chances are that it'll make a significant contribution. For example, we regard the daily commute to work as a necessary hazard of the job. In the same way, even a sedentary desk-bound post will inevitably involve considerable mental activity. Such jobs also require you to leave your seat every now and then for meetings, coffee or toilet breaks. In other words, there is a degree of activity associated with this demand on our life to earn money to pay bills, and this can be measured in terms of the impact on our health and welfare.

In terms of activity expenditure, WHO suggest all adults should undertake 150 minutes of moderate physical activity per week, broken down into five 30-minute sessions plus two days featuring strength exercises. From the age of sixty-five onwards, the weekly requirement rises to 300 minutes of moderate physical activity. This takes the typical age of retirement into account, so you can begin to see the impact employment can have on your health. All too often we talk about work stress, which is a legitimate concern, and yet rarely do we register that having a job (and the physical exertion it demands) can in fact be *good* for your health.

Should you buy into the concept of retirement as a period of gentle leisure, and make no provision to compensate for the loss of employment as well as the mental and physical inactivity, the results could be devastating. Recent studies on the 60–69 age group, which we generally consider to be retired, revealed that typically they spent just fifteen minutes a day in moderate to vigorous physical activity. By contrast, this group spent over eight hours a day in sedentary behaviour. In terms of general health, such a lifestyle is likely to cause problems. Already, 40 per cent of those sixty and over take five or more medications per day.

All is not lost, however. If you're in this age group, or recognise that you're drifting towards a retirement defined by doing very little, now is the time to take action. With the steady loss of muscle mass in mind, it would be advisable to determine your sport participation and/or a training plan not later than the age of about sixty. Remember, lifelong intensive physical activity is essential for healthy ageing. The decisions you take between the ages of sixty and sixty-five will have a profound effect on the rest of your life.

65–74: Second adolescence

Your teenage years are in the distant past, but at sixty-five you face another period of soul-searching, experimentation and boundary testing as you get to grips with your new place in life. Retirement is responsible here. You might have gone from being in charge of a large team in a pressured environment to fetching the milk from your local newsagent. It's a big change, and not always positive, and yet if you don't act quickly a degenerative routine can settle in. Before you know it, you've reached your mid-seventies and those ambitions you harboured on first claiming your pension have withered like your health.

If we were to define this age group by their entrepreneurial endeavours, the results are troubling. Here, the number of startups is suddenly reduced from 26 per cent to only 7 per cent. In my view, this is largely due to the trauma of calling time on work. We're talking about entering a sudden period of inactivity, in the wake of a career, and the impact this can have not just on your physical health but your mental welfare. From first-hand experience, I know how it can press upon your confidence. It can make it very challenging should you decide to return to the workplace, but not impossible.

For financial reasons, given our extended lifespans, you should consider working for seven years beyond the age of retirement. For health reasons, it seems that you should work longer still. In reality, the promised paradise of a work-free life is a desert of despair. The lack of mental and physical stimulus takes its toll on your mind and body. Of those aged sixty-five and over, a significant percentage have one or more chronic diseases. Sadly, and inevitably, training in this age group is directed at the prevention and/or treatment of disease.

On the other hand, this group has very special characteristics. The concept of 'active ageing' is often encouraged here, and promotes endurance exercises such as Nordic walking or cycling. It isn't as effective as mid- to high-intensity workouts or resistance training in terms of building muscle mass, but you will still find it has benefits. Even if you have lost 20 to 40 per cent of your muscle mass, this can be rebuilt at the age of seventy – through appropriate exercise – more easily than in almost any other age group. Studies suggest that at this age we seem to have a genetic disposition that enables us to build muscle more easily than those fifty years younger. After twenty-two weeks of heavy resistance training, for example, men aged 60–71 had positively increased muscle mass and strength to levels comparable with 28–31-year-olds undergoing the same regime.

To understand what's going on here, I'd like to introduce you to myostatin, which is a negative regulator of your skeletal muscle. When myostatin gene expression levels are high, loss of muscle mass will occur. In studies, young men with an average age of twenty-one were compared to men with an average age of sixty-six. After resistance exercise, the older men had lower levels of myostatin and higher levels of folliostatin, which is a positive regulator of muscle mass. In conclusion, men in this age group have a more favourable physiological capacity for muscle growth than younger men.

It's regrettable that this phenomenon, which could have a profound effect on the training of the aged, has been ignored, inadequately utilised and insufficiently explored. I suspect that yet again this is down to the fact that the number of healthy subjects over the age of seventy is too small to conduct any substantial research! We can only hope this situation changes through growing awareness that lost muscle mass can be replaced, and at a time when people wrongly assume that falling apart is a necessary part of the ageing process.

75–84: Late adulthood

By 2050, it's estimated, the percentage of the population aged eighty and over will have increased by a quarter. That's a huge upswing, and yet statistics show that is the age we're at our most inactive and prone to disease. In effect, without a strategy for successful ageing, we're simply shuffling into decrepitude.

At this age, vigorous activity is typically reduced to only five to six minutes a day and sedentary behaviour increased to over nine hours in the same period. That's a lot of time spent staring at the wall, and a depressing picture to paint for those heading into this age bracket.

In addition, loss of muscle mass of between 30 and 60 per cent is a serious problem and the major cause of disability. In my opinion, the loss at this age is so significant that resistance or endurance training will not provide significant improvement. Even strength training will not combat sarcopenia here, as the muscle wastage is too great. Generally, occupational therapy for this age range focuses on improving limited mobility. All is not lost, of course, but I would always recommend commencing an appropriate programme of muscle building at the earliest opportunity.

85–95: Old but not out

Like the category preceding it, very little indeed is known about this age group. Researchers strive for more knowledge. Unfortunately, fit and healthy subjects pushing into their nineties are not easy to find in sufficient numbers.

My personal observation suggests that a 'mid-age crisis' can occur at about the age of eighty-five. Once you reach this stage in life, often with failing health, it can be hard to know what's in store. Even with a successful ageing strategy the future doesn't always look bright. To my mind, this is the category that needs our support and attention, because it's never too late to reclaim quality of life, and with it everything from a sense of independence to wellbeing.

To illustrate this, a 2005 study of a group of ninety-year-old nursing home residents proved that after fourteen weeks of strength training – with two training sessions per week using exercise machines – impressive advances could be made. On average, members of the group lost 3lb of fat while adding 4lb of lean muscle. They increased leg strength by 80 per cent, upper body strength by 40 per cent and joint flexibility by 30 per cent.

Not only is this an incredible physical improvement over a short space of time, the quality of life for these residents would have improved immeasurably. What's more, it reduced the yearly cost of care by $40,000, which was two and a half times the cost of the exercise machines used for the experiment. Even at this advanced age, physical activity can not only help with prevention and cure but offers huge cost savings.

By now, I hope you're beginning to get a sense of where you are in life. It isn't as simple as just asking how old you are. Age and ability don't always go hand in hand, after all. I count myself as a man in his late nineties who is quite capable of outperforming someone twenty years younger in certain strength and flexibility exercises. This isn't down to 'good genes', as is often levelled at me. I have worked hard to achieve the mind and body I possess today, and just hope that my example can serve as an incentive. It is, I hope, a positive means of assessing the prospect of successful ageing. The alternative is to consider the fact that physical and mental inactivity is one of the major causes of disease, death and huge financial costs.

Whichever way you look at it, you owe it to yourself to take the next step.

Evaluating your health and wellbeing

For each result that says you should start or continue an activity or exercise programme in this section you should only do so under close supervision of your doctor.

If you've reached this point having decided to make a change, then congratulations! In many ways, you've overcome the hardest part of the process. Ahead of any competitive race, whether it's on the water or the track, I find that moment before the starter's gun can be nerve-racking. That's why it's so important to be fully aware of your capabilities at this point. It'll give you control and confidence moving forward, and it begins with a thorough assessment of your physical and mental welfare.

So, following our exercise to raise awareness of age and ability, what we have next is a series of questions concerning your health and wellbeing. I have devised these with Sylvia to help you determine your current level of fitness within the context of your lifestyle and – under supervision from your doctor – help you to establish an appropriate action plan.

All you have to do is answer the questions openly and honestly.

No.	Question	☹✋	☹	😐	☺	☺💧
1 Your Organic Risk Factors						
1	How high is your blood pressure?	Very high risk	High	Raised	Normal	Optimal
	Do you know your values?	≥180/≥110	160–179/ 100–109	140–159/ 90–99	130–139/ 85–89	≤130/≤85
2	Have you had one of the following illnesses?	More than once	Once	Slightly	Little	None
	Heart attack					
	Stroke					
	Heart operation					
	Cardiac arrhythmia					
3	Breathing difficulties	Acute	Chronic	Allergic	None	None
4	Vascular disease/ venous weakness	Very high	High	Medium	Low	None
5	Diabetes type 1/2	Very high	High	Medium	Low	None
6	Thyroid over and under function	Very high	High	Medium	Low	None
7	Obesity/overweight	Very High	High	Medium	Low	None
8	Osteoporosis	Very High	High	Medium	Low	None
9	Fibromyalgia	Very High	High	Medium	Low	None
10	Kidney disease	Very High	High	Medium	Low	None
11	Cancer	Very High	High	Medium	Low	None
	Totals					

© Sylvia Gattiker

Results:

- Only ☺/☺👍 You are set to start a fitness programme, or develop the one you're on.

- More than 7 ☺/☺/☺👍 You can start a fitness programme, but build up slowly.

- More than 6 ☺ You can start a fitness programme, but only one for beginners.

- More than 3 ☹ Consult your doctor before starting any exercise.programme.

If you marked any of the questions with ☹🖐 then it's important to see your doctor immediately. Don't panic. Just be sure to work closely with your GP in dealing with any underlying health issues.

2 Your Musculoskeletal System						
No.	Question	☹🖐	☹	☺	☺	☺👍
1	Do you have backache?	Very strong and permanent	Strong and very often/often	Quite strong and regularly	Rarely	Never
2	Do you have scoliosis?	Acute	Strongly	A little	None	None
3	Do you have or have you had a slipped disk?	Acute	Yes, often	Yes, but a while ago	Yes, but it's healed	Never

4	Do you have displaced vertebrae?	Acute	Somewhat	Slight	None	None
5	Do you have M. Scheuermann, M. Bechtorow, spondyloses?	Acute	Yes	Slight	None	None
6	Do you have osteoarthritis?	Acute	Strong	Slight	A little	None
7	Do you have arthritis?	Acute	Chronic	Occasionally	A little	None
8	Do you have rheumatism?	Acute	Chronic	Occasionally	A little	None
9	Do you have movement limitations and pain in any of the following ?	Acute	Strong	Somewhat	Slight	None
	Shoulder					
	Elbow					
	Forearm/hand					
	Hip					
	Knee					
	Foot					
	Totals					

© Sylvia Gattiker

Results:

- Only ☺/☺👍 You are set to start a fitness programme, or develop the one you're on.

- More than 7 ☺/☺/☺👍 You can start a fitness programme, but build up slowly.

- More than 6 ☺ You can start a fitness programme, but only one for beginners.

- More than 3 ☹ Consult your doctor before starting any exercise programme.

Once again, if you've answered any questions as ☹✋ then check in with your doctor at the earliest opportunity.

3 Your Medication						
No.	Question	☹✋	☹	☺	☺	☺👍
1	Blood pressure regulating	High dose	Yes	Small dose	Previously but no longer	None
2	Circulation regulating	High dose	Yes	Small dose	Previously but no longer	None
3	Heart stimulants	High dose	Yes	Small dose	Previously but no longer	None
4	Diuretics	High dose	Yes	Small dose	Previously but no longer	None
5	Respiratory	High dose	Yes	Small dose	Previously but no longer	None
6	Diabetes medication or insulin	High dose	Yes	Small dose	Previously but no longer	None
7	Painkillers	High dose	Yes	Small dose	Previously but no longer	None
8	Psychiatric	High dose	Yes	Small dose	Previously but no longer	None

9	Blood thinner	High dose	Yes	Small dose	Previously but no longer	None
10	Other medication	High dose	Yes	Small dose	Previously but no longer	None
	Totals					

© Sylvia Gattiker

Results:

- Only ☺/☺👍 You are set to start a fitness programme, or develop the one you're on.

- More than 7 😐/☺/☺👍 You can start a fitness programme, but build up slowly.

- More than 6 😐 You can start a fitness programme, but only one for beginners.

- More than 3 ☹ Please make sure you see your doctor before attempting any exercise programme.

If any of your answers consist of ☹✋ then see your doctor. They can monitor and review any medication course you might be taking.

4 General Health and Activity						
No.	Question	☹✋	☹	😐	☺	☺👍
1	Do you suffer from one or more chronic illnesses?	More than 3	2–3	1	None	None
2	Have you been regularly ill in the last couple of years?	More than 4 times	3–4	1–2	Maybe a cold	No
3	Rate your cholesterol level	Very High	High	Slightly raised	Normal	Excellent
4	Do you or did you smoke?	More than 20 per day	20 per day	A few a day	I've stopped	Never
5	Waist size (in centimetres)					
	Female	> 98	> 88	> 80	under 80	under 75
	Male	> 112	> 102	> 94	under 94	under 89
6	How well can you climb stairs?	I can't	Very badly	Slowly and it's difficult	No problem	Easy
7	Can you get out of a chair?	I need help	I need to support myself	Slowly and it's difficult	No problem	Easy
8	Can you balance on one leg?	No	No	With help	Yes	Easy
9	Can you stand up with your eyes shut for 30 seconds?	No	No	Less than 30 seconds	Yes	More than 30 seconds
10	How often do you exercise for more than 30 minutes at a time (walking, swimming, jogging, riding a bike)?	Never	Rarely	Once a week	2–3 times a week	Daily
11	Do you have to take a break if you're on your feet for more than 30 minutes?	Very often	Often	At least once	Never	Never
12	Can you move without help?	No, I have a wheelchair	No, I have a walker	No, I use a stick	Yes	Yes
	Totals					

© Sylvia Gattiker

Results:

- Only ☺/☺👍 Well done and keep going!

- More than 7 ☺/☺👍 You're heading in the right direction. Keep doing what you're doing and build up to an even healthier lifestyle.

- More than 7 ☺ You should start an activity and movement programme – but only one for beginners – and aim to lead a healthier lifestyle.

- More than 3 ☹ It's time to review your lifestyle. Try to be more active and healthier.

If ☹✋ appears in your answers then make an appointment to see your doctor. They can review your health and devise an appropriate plan to improve it.

No.	Question	☹🖐	☹	😐	☺	☺👍
	**5 Sleep Cycle/Psyche**					
1	Do you sleep well?	Only with tablets	Very badly	Sometimes	Yes	Yes
2	Do you sleep all the way through the night?	Only with tablets	Very badly	I wake up once or twice	Yes	Yes
3	How long do you normally sleep?	Less than 4 hours	4–5 hours	6 hours	7 hours	More than 7 hours
4	Do you regularly go to bed before midnight?	Never	Rarely	Occasionally	Always	Always
5	Your personal environment					
	I live in a partnership (married/civil partnership/ life partner)	Very unhappily	Unhappily	I've got used to the situation	I'm satisfied	Happy
	I live alone	Very unhappily	Unhappily	I've got used to the situation	I'm satisfied	Happy
6	Are you worried (e.g. about the future)?	Very strongly	Strongly	Quite a lot	A little	No
7	Are you depressive?	Very strongly	Strongly	Sometimes	A little	No
8	Are you often bored?	Always	Very often	Sometimes	A little	Never
9	Do you have problems with your memory?	Very often	Often	Sometimes	A little	Never
10	Are you happy with your life?	Not at all	No	Often	Always	Always

© Sylvia Gattiker

Results:

- Only ☺/☺👍 You are a happy and grounded person – keep going and stay active!

- More than 6 ☺/☺👍 You are basically happy and have a good sleep cycle. Remember, movement and activity underpin your lifestyle and successful ageing!

- More than 6 ☺ Try to find a positive attitude to your life. Take part in group activities and maintain regular exercise.

- More than 3 ☹ Consider opening up about any issues on your mind. Also address any sleep problems you may be experiencing.

If ☹✋ features in any of your answers then consult your doctor. Your mental health is as important to them as your physical welfare, and help is always available.

No.	Question	☹🤚	☹	😐	😊	😊💧
6 Diet						
1	Do you value a healthy diet?	I don't pay any attention	No	Rarely	Most of the time	Always
2	How many portions of fruit and vegetables do you eat per day?	None	1–2	3	4–5	More than 5
3	Do you eat lots of sweet things?	Almost exclusively	Several times a day	Often (several times a week)	Rarely	Never
4	Do you often eat fast food?	Almost exclusively	Several times a day	Often (several times a week)	Rarely	Never
5	Do you eat lots of bread?	Almost exclusively	Several times a day	Often (several times a week)	Rarely	Never
6	Do you eat lots of pasta?	Almost exclusively	Several times a day	Often (several times a week)	Rarely	Never
7	Do you often eat out?	Exclusively	Almost always	Often (several times a week)	Rarely	Never
8	Do you eat regularly?	No	No	Rarely	Mostly	Always
9	How much do you drink (unsweetened, non-alcoholic drinks)?	Less than ½ litre per day	Less than 1 litre per day	About 1 litre a day	1½ litres per day	More than 1½ litres per day
10	Do you drink alcohol?	Regularly, a lot and spirits	A lot, and spirits	Daily and sometimes spirits	1–2 glasses of wine per day	Never
	Totals					

© Sylvia Gattiker

Results:

- Only ☺/☺👍 Bravo!

- More than 6 ☺/☺👍 You are feeding yourself healthily. Paired with a fitness or movement programme you are on your way to a successful old age and a healthy lifestyle!

- More than 6 ☹/😐 You should think about reviewing your eating and drinking habits.

- More than 1 ☹🖐 This indicates a high risk to your health. Your doctor can help you to establish a healthy eating plan.

Now enter the total values of the individual results into the table on the next page. Finally add each column to provide your results total.

Total results		☹✋	☹	😐	☺	☺👍
No.						
1	Result Table 1					
2	Result Table 2					
3	Result Table 3					
4	Result Table 4					
5	Result Table 5					
6	Result Table 6					
RESULT TOTALS:						

© Sylvia Gattiker

Evaluation of your results:

Only ☺/☺👍 You're already on the right track. Stay as active as you are and keep taking part in life. For you, there are no risks to starting a fitness programme!

More than 38 ☺/☺👍 You are well on the way to an active and successful old age. Your lifestyle is health ori-entated. You can start with a fitness programme if you are not doing one already. If you are starting a programme, begin slowly and build it up over a period of time.

More than 38 😐 You need to change your lifestyle. Focus more on your diet and exercise more. You could start an exercise programme, but only at beginners' level.

More than 38 ☹ It's always worth seeing your doctor before beginning any exercise plan. In this case it's important to work with a medical professional in establishing a safe way to improve your health and welfare.

More than 1 ☹✋ Consider this to be a health wake-up call. It's not too late to make changes for the better, but check in with your GP first.

Next steps

By getting you to complete these questionnaires, with an awareness of your age and ability, I hope to have awakened a desire in you to change. From minor adjustments to major upheavals, we all approach the future according to how we've lived our lives. At the same time, we exist in a society that prepares every one of us for the same outcome – retirement. But as you head towards that moment, have you ever stopped to wonder if the reality will meet your expectations?

Chances are you've worked hard throughout your life this far. In that time, you've paid into your pension pot, and now you're looking forward to the day you can 'put your feet up'. My question is, what will you do once you've grown tired of doing nothing?

Life for me, even now, is extremely positive. This is entirely down to the fact that I made the changes I'm encouraging you to consider. So, rather than view later life as being your sunset years, look at it as a new dawn.

195

By rebuilding your body through diet and exercise, creating a purpose through work and rejuvenating your mind in the process, you too can discover what I have found.

To sum it up, I find being very old most enjoyable! I don't believe that I am abnormal. To you I may seem like an exotic ape from the primeval forest. In reality, I am a perfectly normal person, free from additives, drugs, performance-enhancing substances or anything of that ilk. For me, as it should be for you, being old is a privilege. At my age, there are so many things I have experienced it seems that history repeats itself and I am wiser for it.

Even if you've arrived at this point feeling reasonably fit and healthy, I urge you to think ahead and plan for your future as I have. It might seem unconventional. Those lifestyle hoardings for retirement homes don't yet show old-timers like me pumping iron in the gym, for example, but I am living proof that it brings far greater rewards than just a toned body. I suppose there are things that you might not be able to do any longer, but aside from rowing I haven't found many so far. In fact, I have found successful ageing to be a wonderful, rich, engaging and fulfilling experience that goes way beyond the bleak reality of traditional retirement. So, having established a sense of where you are in life, let's look at how the three components of successful ageing can help to build a brighter future.

15

Work for Life

I am keenly aware that I face a challenge in promoting the virtues of working into later life. I am just one very old man who has demonstrated the virtues of successful ageing, and yet I am up against an entire industry that depends on selling you the concept of retirement as a thirty-year paid holiday.

We have seen, from my experience and in statistics and research, that inactivity is closely associated with ill health, while our extended lifespans have rendered the pension model unfit for purpose. Quite simply, something has to be done, and yet I know full well that it appears as if I am advocating the removal of a carrot and its replacement with a stick. In practice, however, regular work in later life can come as a liberation.

Often, throughout our careers, work can feel like a chore. We're slaves to a mortgage, with growing families who depend on us to pay the bills and put food on the table. But as the years pass, and our children grow up, so I believe that work can take on a new purpose. It just happens to take shape at a time when we're conditioned to expect a payoff for our hard labours in the form of a cosy retirement. It's no wonder that people look forward to this moment, and even give up work early for an easy life of golf and long cruises.

In reality, however, a holiday at sea won't take up thirty years of your time, while trundling along the fairway in an electric buggy will do little for your fitness. Before you know it that dream has turned to tedium, while any plans you might have had are overshadowed by ill health. This might be an extreme scenario, but if you can register that a kernel of truth exists within it then all of a sudden the prospect of a return to work can feel rejuvenating.

The question of what you can do in terms of employment is not easy to answer. So much depends on your personal situation in terms of health, fitness and finances. I believe all three are inextricably linked, in that work brings an income while keeping you occupied and in shape (if underpinned with a muscle-building programme). Often, it's a question of taking small steps back into the workplace, or even setting up an enterprise that gives you complete control.

Then there is the issue of the nature of the work you consider to be attractive. Again, everyone comes to this with a different outlook. You might once have been a CEO, with no intention of going back to the level of responsibility and pressure you once shouldered, and that's fine. There's nothing stopping you from picking up manual work, for example, which could prove to be a childhood dream come true. As we've seen, older generations are often the most enterprising. Even if you've passed your fifties, it's not too late to apply your wealth of knowledge and experience to a startup. Nobody is saying it'll be easy. Establishing a new business can be demanding. It can involve reaching out to forge new contacts and opportunities, and take up a great deal of time and energy. At a stage of life when your high point has become an afternoon quiz show on television, what a wonderful opportunity this could be! It's a question of embracing the fact that we might have numerous jobs throughout our lives. Not only does this allow us to extend the period in which we consider ourselves to be useful, by continuing to make a valuable contribution to society we can only feel better about ourselves. What's more, with work come opportunities . . .

From a personal standpoint, and quite without design, I now find my services are in demand as someone who embodies successful ageing. Since my mid-eighties, in fact, when I woke up to the perils of retirement and the possibilities in later life associated with building muscle, I have never been busier! Following the end of my post as ambassador for a chain of gyms, I have gone on to give lectures and speaking engagements around the world. I am often asked to provide media interviews, and always seize the opportunity to share and discuss my views on radio, television and the Internet. I was flown to the States to film an 'infomercial' about a juicer, and even presented a TEDx talk that has amassed well over half a million views. I find the work varied, enjoyable and stimulating. It's a pleasure, never a chore, and brings benefits that go way beyond financial reward.

So, what I'm encouraging you to do here is fundamentally change your attitude to working after the age of retirement. It doesn't have to be a necessary evil, but can be an opportunity that brings benefits beyond a salary to supplement what might be a breadline income. Even if you're comfortable on your pension, and thankful for the annuity that you purchased before living until a grand old age, just think of the pressure you'll be taking away from the younger generation to pay for it. It might not seem like much, but if everyone shared the same approach it could benefit society as a whole.

The possibilities are endless. In a nutshell, it's a question of regarding retirement not as an end game but a new beginning. Where you take this aspect of successful ageing from here is entirely up to you.

16

Nutrition for Life

The fact is we live in an age in which we consume more food than we need. By eating less, or improving our nutrition, we stand a better chance of living healthier lives, and that extends to our later years. On this note, it's critical to stress that the concept of an appropriate diet is down to the individual, their health and lifestyle, as well as factors such as the degree of exercise they undertake each day. All manner of variables come into play here, in fact, which is why it's so important to review your eating habits with a medical professional. Only they can make an informed opinion as to whether you need to make changes, and effectively put your health first.

From a personal perspective, when I've needed to improve my diet (to lose weight, for example) I begin by writing down my reasons. Next I ask myself if this is the best time to make such changes. Before I commence, for about a week I keep a record of everything I eat and drink as well as a diary of my activities in that time. This helps me to identify problem areas, and what I most want to change. Finally, I make sure I am in the right frame of mind to see it through. Motivation is vital here, so it's worth taking time to identify a goal you really want to achieve.

To begin, in a bid to be realistic, I choose two or three small changes I can make to my diet. Next I put together an action plan to follow with clear targets. When I feel I've succeeded I move on to more changes or build on the ones I have already established. I have always set myself clear goals, but it's not just about my weight on the scales. Losing inches from my waist helps to lower the risk of conditions like type 2 diabetes and high blood pressure.

I don't forget to add exercise to the mix, of course, and indeed Sylvia won't let me! Doing more not only helps me burn more calories but keeps me busy and content. In terms of getting into shape, we now know that a specified training regime requires specific nutrition. For example, endurance training would require more carbohydrates including carbohydrate loading. Muscle building would require a protein-rich diet with protein supplements and certain amino acids, especially for those of advanced age.

Now I have no intention of being prescriptive about what you can and cannot eat. I believe it's a question of being aware of *everything* you're eating, from the enjoyment it brings to the purpose it serves. In striking a balance, food should always be a pleasurable feature of your daily routine without compromising your health. For this reason I recommend a balanced diet including the following foods:

- bread, potatoes and other cereals

- fruits and vegetables

- meat, fish, eggs and alternatives such as pulses and nuts

- dairy products

- healthy fats such as monounsaturated fatty acids (MUFAs), found in nuts, olives and avocados, and fish rich in omega-3s.

In considering your relationship with food, and following consultation with your doctor, I hope to seed a change in later life that might go some way towards improving a grave situation – not just for you as an individual but society as a whole.

My later life in action

In my general diet, no single food contains all the nutrients that I need to stay healthy. So the golden rule is that I eat a variety of foods each day. Eating healthily does not mean cutting out foods I enjoy, but simply eating some foods less often and/or in smaller portions, and eating more of other foods.

Usually I start the day with a healthy breakfast; by doing this I find it much easier to control my weight. Then throughout the day I eat regular, balanced meals. I try to have meals at planned times during the day and aim to include at least five portions of fresh fruit and vegetables each day. In practice, I have some at every meal and I only half fill my plate with vegetables or salad and divide the other half between meat, fish, eggs or beans and carbohydrates like potatoes or rice. I always try to choose foods and drinks that are low in sugar and avoid snacks where possible.

Very importantly, it takes time for my brain to know my stomach is full. So I wait at least 5–10 minutes before deciding if I need to eat any more. I watch my portion sizes, especially when eating out, and avoid eating at the same time as doing something else. Grazing while working, reading or watching TV simply means you're at risk of not paying attention to a vital fuel stop. Instead, I eat slowly and really taste what I am putting in my mouth.

In addition, I have cut down on salty foods. Salt is essential for health but eating too much of it increases your risk of high blood pressure and stroke. I check the labels on foods such as processed meats, savoury snacks, biscuits, cheese, bacon, some soups and ready meals – much of the salt we eat is already in food when we buy it. So remember, always think before you sprinkle salt on your meal. At the same time, it may surprise some to learn that I do not rigidly avoid food high in animal or vegetable fat. This is a recent development for me, however, and a reflection of my enthusiasm for keeping abreast of current scientific research into nutrition in later life. My diet is something I appraise closely and evolve where supported by evidence-based findings.

As for dealing with dietary issues that affect many people my age, I find that bran should only be used as a last resort to prevent constipation. First, I make sure that I have enough wholegrain cereals and fruit in my diet. Drinking plenty of liquids can help too and physical activity helps keep bowels moving! Since I began adding linseed to my diet, my digestion has been perfect.

Staying hydrated is as important to me as making sure I'm eating sensibly. For one thing, it reduces the chances of constipation as well as effectively keeping us alive! I drink plenty of fluid, usually about 6–8 cups each day, but don't restrict myself to water. I prefer green tea but you may choose coffee, fruit juice or squash, which are equally good. I find it particularly important to drink plenty in hot weather and after I have trained or exercised.

When it comes to fuelling my workouts, I always take a protein shake after training. This consists of whey protein and amino acids including leucine, the amino acid used in the biosynthesis of proteins. It's important that the post-training shake is consumed within thirty minutes of the end of the session.

It's also worth noting that I don't drink alcohol unless I'm out for the evening. Then, it's a glass of champagne (and nothing else!). Essentially, I always try to moderate my alcohol intake. It's high in calories and dissolves good intentions.

Finally, I'd like to stress that eating remains a great pleasure in my life as I strive for successful ageing. I don't feel as if I deprive myself of treats. I find pleasure in eating sensibly and in the health benefits that come from this when combined with an active life and physical exercise. To give you a flavour, here's a menu from a typical day in my life:

Breakfast

2 bananas, grapefruit

Peaches, pineapple or kiwi fruit, according to season and availability.

Porridge, cooked with water and milk.

I also take an Omega 3 capsule and vitamin D, and a whey protein drink

Lunch

Either smoked mackerel or a vegetable drink.

I may also eat cheese – Tilsiter mild or camembert are my favourites. If I have expended a lot of energy training, I will eat more.

Dinner

Meat or fish and two vegetables plus beans or lentils. The beans and lentils are valuable vegetable protein.

No dessert.

Essentially, this is my typical daily diet. I don't make wholesale changes when I'm training (apart from a bowl of pasta after resistance work when I need to replenish my carbohydrate reserves) but what works for me may not work for you. In addition, Sylvia and I are continuously exploring new eating plans and different training regimes. I consider it to be flexible, and simply aim to eat so I can live life to the best of my abilities.

17

Exercise for Life

From an early age, we're encouraged to be active. We live in an age of obesity, and so any drive to get people off the sofa has to be a good thing. At the same time, I'm struck by how the message changes when we reach a certain age. Post-retirement, we're almost expected to slow down. Instead of vigorous exercise or high intensity workouts, our focus is turned to the prospect of gently bobbing to music in the shallow end of the swimming pool or simply enjoying fresh air as if somehow that will magically rejuvenate us.

Now, any form of physical activity is a good thing in my opinion, and I'm well aware that we all have different abilities depending on our health at the time. But

I do hold that by leaving older people to feel they have no right to push beyond light exercise, we are doing our society a great disservice. To illustrate my point, have you ever heard of advanced training regimes for the 80-plus age group? It might seem outlandish to some, but with so much attention paid to getting younger people fit for life we're allowing the older generation to languish.

In the course of our working relationship, Sylvia and I have focused on establishing and refining a training programme for people over seventy. We believe ourselves to be unique in what we are doing. But why should it be up to us to do this? Surely it should be the responsibility of health groups and governments to invest in the research that is required to get results. The efforts of a nonagenarian and his sixty-something coach look paltry in comparison to what could be done, and yet if you'll consider me to be a work in progress then the results speak volumes.

In my experience, any kind of physical exercise should aim to develop and maintain strength, stamina, flexibility and balance. Strength is critical in muscle building, which is key to combating sarcopenia. Stamina helps you to walk any distance, swim and mow the lawn, while strength helps you carry shopping or get out of a chair. Flexibility helps you to bend, climb into a car, wash your hair and get dressed. Balance helps you to walk and climb steps confidently, stand from a sitting position, and respond quickly if you trip. Combined, these assets effectively allow us to lead our lives.

It should also be stressed that exercise is a loose term, and we often perform it without realising! In effect, it embraces everything from activity in the workplace, including the commute, to specific workouts or a sporting pursuit. With retirement, of course, work may no longer be part of the equation. For older people this simply reduces the opportunity to be active, which is all the more reason to think about your routine.

If you are generally fit and have no health conditions that limit your ability to move around, it's recommended that you should build up to doing two and a half hours of moderate aerobic activity each week. This can include walking fast, cycling on level ground or even pushing a lawnmower. Just try not to rely too heavily on everyday activities, such as shopping and housework, as they don't increase your heart rate as effectively as specific exercise. If you are already active, you can improve your fitness and health by doing seventy-five minutes of vigorous activity during the week such as running, cycling fast, climbing stairs, playing tennis or dancing.

While maintaining an appropriate level of activity is a foundation for successful ageing, our main finding is that muscle mass is critical – but not just in terms of physical strength. Through the movement, usage and action of our muscles, messenger substances are produced which increase hormone production including testosterone (the 'youth' hormone). Indeed, exercise can have a profound positive effect on the brain. It's even been linked to the prevention or delay of cognitive function loss and neurodegenerative disease. Simply by following an informed muscle-building training programme, old age can become a time of rejuvenation, and I speak from experience.

Muscle-strengthening exercises include lifting weights (including moving heavy loads such as your shopping), doing sit-ups, dancing, heavy gardening and yoga. Your muscles have no biological watch. In fact, they're completely renewed every fifteen years regardless of exercise, but that does not mean they're strong. We need to help them along by doing exercises and maintaining an active lifestyle.

Sylvia and I have found that specially adapted training regimes, together with diet modifications, can still build muscle in extreme old age. As disease and physical degeneration is often a factor for people in this category, any plan should always be accompanied by extensive diagnostic tests and constant re-evaluation. Nevertheless, we have demonstrated that a standard of fitness can be achieved in an amazingly short period of time that was previously thought impossible. Devising a training routine that works for you can enable you to achieve results that are both wide-ranging and life-enhancing. In putting together a safe, appropriate routine that builds muscle, you'll find improvements in everything from cardiovascular health, to endurance, stamina and strength, to flexibility, power, speed, coordination, balance and agility.

In considering what a difference such a transformation could make to your later life, we must recognise that exercise can no longer be seen as a lifestyle option when it comes to our later years. It is *essential*, in my view, on a personal level and for our wider society.

Understanding exercise

Physical activity leads to a healthy body. This is an indisputable fact. It was formulated by Hippocrates (460–377 BC) who said, 'all functional body parts, when stimulated by physical activity, develop well, remain healthy, and age at a slower pace.' However, it's important to stress that physical activity and physical exercise are not one and the same thing. There are different kinds of physical activity, such as work-related activity, activity related to housekeeping, and leisure-related activity. These activities are all undertaken for specific purposes. You might have to get to work on time, tidy the house before visitors arrive or enjoy a morning in the park with your grandchildren. Physical exercise is very different, in that our goal is to improve our fitness.

In order to get fit, we perform *repetitions* – which means undertaking the same movement a certain number of times without a break. This is known as a *set*. For example, squats with fifteen repetitions in two sets means 2 × 15 repetitions, with a short break between sets. Normally, a break is measured as the time required for you to take ten breaths (to a maximum of thirty seconds).

Repetitions, carried out in sets, are designed as super-threshold activities that take you close to the limits of performance and exhaustion. The number of repetitions, the resistance, the type and speed of movement all affect the results. Through this kind of exercise, the body reacts with functional adaptations. As a result, you can attain an improvement of your physical and psychological state. That's why it's necessary to perform any exercise in your fitness routine correctly and in every training session, and always try to increase the number of repetitions or the *intensity*.

This describes the level at which performing an exercise can be made more difficult, typically by increasing weight, resistance, the range of motion or number of repetitions without a break. Also slow the speed of the exercise, which puts more strain on your muscles, or place a cushion under your supporting foot to make balancing more difficult.

Additionally, through the increase of the repetitions or intensity of an exercise, you will find that an improvement in health-related bodily fitness is attainable. While increasing the number of repetitions improves endurance and raising intensity boosts strength, what really matters for your health here is your total energy consumption. This is the sum of physical activity, which combines both exercise and the tasks you carry out as part of day-to-day life.

A great deal depends on individual factors when it comes to working out your desired total volume of physical activity and physical exercise. That is why the exercise recommendations we have listed in the pages that follow are of a general nature. In every case, it should be said, frequent physical activity or exercise is necessary for the attainment of any health-related benefits. How you react to training is down to a combination of genetics and how long, how often and how consistently you carry it out. Depending on the type of exercise, also be sure to build rest and recovery periods into your regime. Not only does this reduce the chances of injury, it's the time when muscles grow and develop. Some bodybuilders are convinced that this occurs at night. As brilliant as that might be – essentially acquiring a beach-ready physique from the comfort of your bed – there is no scientific proof for this. So unless research proves otherwise, you can consider the downtime between exercise days as a chance for your body to go to work, rather than when you hit the pillow at night.

Finally, I can't stress enough that devising any physical exercise routine in later life should be undertaken in conjunction with your doctor. They will have a clear understanding of your health and abilities, and will be able to advise you on a sensible plan that makes your welfare a priority at all times.

So, with your GP's blessing, the next question is: where do you go to work out?

The problems and possibilities of the gym

While the rise of the gym as a public space should be welcomed, I always feel that more could be done to accommodate the older generation. It can be intimidating for anyone to walk through those doors for the first time, but it's especially tough if you feel you're going to be the oldest person present by twenty years or more.

In addition, research has shown that older people prefer to train in groups of their own age. If the fitness industry could just recognise this, they'd find a huge and largely untapped market. Membership could in certain cases, as in Japan, be restricted to those above seventy, or have an off-peak membership for the elderly. Ideally, in a bid to connect and lead by example, the coaches would be of the same age group. As well as providing suitable exercise plans, and overseeing their implementation, they could make their assessments available to the individual's doctor where appropriate to provide holistic support with measurable results in both health and welfare. In taking this model further, I believe a gym workout could become part of the patient's medical history, treatment and healthcare programme.

Certainly treatment of disease by exercise is receiving more attention by the medical profession, but I feel further steps can be taken in terms of cooperation with gyms and health clubs. In an ideal world, we would see a close working partnership between all sectors of the fitness industry and the medical profession. The fact is that many gyms tend to focus on helping clients improve their physical appearance rather than their overall health. While exercise is recognised by the medical profession to be both a prevention and cure, as most commonly seen in physiotherapy practice, I feel the fitness sector has not fully risen to the challenge. Even though doing a very modest amount of exercise can produce dramatic results, it hasn't been enough to persuade doctors to prescribe time in the gym by default as a viable tool to improve health.

As exercise treatment is long term, the medical profession is justified in being sceptical of the fitness industry. Doctors use evidence-based medicine, after all, and expect their partners to offer evidenced-based treatment. In my opinion, the fitness industry does not produce sufficient statistics or evidence to support any claim that their services tangibly improve health. Figures are one thing, but we only have to look at membership behaviour to realise that the fitness indus-try simply isn't working as it should be. The fact is people who sign up to a gym have every chance of just not using their membership or quitting early. Indeed, 30 per cent are said to leave after four months, with just over half of the initial number gone within a year. While people leave for complex reasons, of course, an underlying cause has to be the lack of any significant improvement in their health. The clientele of fitness centres are largely in the 35–55 age group. This group has not lost daily activity energy expenditure as have the retired aged. Muscle building for the inactive older population is more complex, but there are few other options at present for the aged than fitness centres.

The relationship between medicine and the fitness industry has some way to go in order to work in harmony. Meanwhile, academic support for encouraging the elderly to exercise seems almost non-existent. Those with relevant university degrees, e.g. bachelor or master of sport or health science, can rarely be found working in a gym, which is why I regard my coach, Sylvia, as one of a kind. She has an academic background in prevention and health management, as well as huge practical experience in training clients. She should be regarded as a shining example of what the fitness industry can offer if it wishes to become a genuine force for good.

In an ideal world, I believe, coaches could be certified with the medical knowledge and skills to treat certain ailments. This might be a long way off, but all progress begins with a vision! The fact is almost all over-65s have one or more chronic diseases. I just hope that the fitness industry will one day work closely with the medical profession and academics to deliver successful ageing for all.

Physical exercise is not the preserve of the young. As

much as disease prevention, it's a key to healthy living that should be available to us all, and I would encourage you to visit your nearest gym and find out what's on offer. If you're worried or uncomfortable in such a new, unfamiliar environment then bring a friend. Gym staff will generally make every effort to accommodate and support you. It really is just a question of asking. And frankly, if more of us express an interest, then in due course the big chains will become more active in embracing our custom.

If you're considering training in a gym, and have your doctor's backing, then I would recommend that you do so under the guidance of a fitness professional. Working out under the watchful eye of a trainer will give you peace of mind and the confidence to know that you're on the right road to getting the results you desire. Joining in as part of a small group can also bring social benefits, as well as reducing the expense. At times, you may well be advised to make small changes and adaptations to your regime in order to attain your goal, and this may include easing off. As tempting as it might be to push on regardless – and this is often the case as you begin to make progress – it's always worth listening to professional advice to avoid injury and continue making long-term advances. Just be aware that for all the critical support you should call upon to make the most of your new exercise regime, only you can turn the changes you desire into a reality.

So, from the age of sixty upwards I would suggest you start to train twice a week with resistance training. You should aim to improve your entire body under supervision by an experienced instructor as well as your doctor. If you have fewer training sessions per week you may not achieve your desired effects, while too many training units per week may put a strain on the body, increase the risk of injury and jeopardise physical improvements.

As you get older (especially from seventy onwards), I recommend incorporating resting phases into your training programme. These phases are designed to give your body a break from physical exertion, and can extend to anything from steam baths and saunas to massages or relaxation exercises. In effect, it's a chance to reward yourself for all your hard work.

Endurance training doesn't have to be confined to the gym. What matters is that you have space to undertake your activity safely, and even enjoy it. Your choice of the kind of activity you do for your endurance training is entirely up to you. All dynamic training forms like walking, jogging, swimming, rowing, hiking or cycling are ideal, and should be carried out in a series of repetitions. If your GP agrees and if you are otherwise reasonably fit and well, I would suggest aiming to perform the same repetition four times over 15 minutes, three times over 20 minutes, or twice over 30 minutes non-stop. As a guide your ideal endurance programme would include six repetitions over 30 minutes, three over 60 minutes, or three over 45 minutes. Also keep in mind that muscular strength training, twice a week, is basic and more important than endurance training.

By pacing yourself depending upon your age and with your doctor's approval, you can use the following broad guidelines to monitor your training intensity:

60–70 years 128–112 pulse beats/minute

70–80 years 120–100 pulse beats/minute

80+ years   112–95 pulse beats/minute

Exercising at home

Despite my belief that the health industry could go further to support the elderly, I would support your efforts to join a gym and work out with a professional trainer. Nevertheless, there's still a great deal you can do at home. Whether you're unable to travel far for health reasons, or simply prefer to exercise in your own space, you still have every chance to put your body (and mind) through its paces. Making sure your GP is on board before you begin, here are some general tips for making the most of what's on offer under your own roof:

- To begin with, look for easy ways to fit more movement into your day-to-day routine. For example, why not stand up when talking on the phone, park a bit further away from your destination or get off the bus a stop earlier?

- Aim to take two steps at a time walking up the stairs and – if appropriate – don't hold on to the banister. This will lengthen your stride and lessen your dependency on your arm strength to pull you up the stairs.

- When you're walking down the stairs, try to hold on to the banister not too hard or not at all. You'll find that your balance and coordination will improve day by day.

- Focus on your posture. Keep your back straight by imagining that you're marching. Swing your arms and take large strides. This will help keep your hips moving, which is very important as we grow older.

- If possible, plan a walk into your day. If this is something you've not done for a while then ask someone in your family, or a friend, to walk with you. Aim to gradually increase the length and speed of your walks to burn more calories.

- To strengthen your arms when you're sitting in your favourite armchair, just use your arms to push yourself up out of the chair and back down again. Do this five times and then take a rest. Then do it again. This way you'll build up your upper body slowly and comfortably!

- Do you have grandchildren? If so, then take them out for a walk to the park. Even if you can't keep up with them, you'll naturally start moving a little bit quicker.

- If you're an early riser, why not go for a brisk morning walk rather than lying in bed? You might even consider taking a couple of ski sticks and doing some Nordic walking.

- Fitness isn't always just your body. Keep your mind fit too. Do the crossword in the paper every day, or a Sudoku or a brainteaser. Anything that stimulates your mind will help, even if it's a hobby such as knitting or model building. And make sure you do this every day. Don't just sit and watch the TV! Learn something new.

- Get creative. Do something different that challenges your mind. It might be painting or writing, or what about a new business venture? Keep abreast of modern technology and trends. Join a sports club, even as a social member, and mix with people of different generations.

- There's no shame in being vain! Take pride in your appearance, look smart. Put on your make-up or have a shave, get your hair done and wear nice clothes. Remember, you're beautiful!

- My advice to gentlemen is to wear braces instead of a belt so that the lower part of the lungs is not constricted. Constriction encourages superficial breathing, which especially in advanced age can lead to an arrhythmic heart rate.

- Trainers should be worn, as you should be ready to sprint to catch your bus, train or tram. Sprinting can greatly increase your level of fitness.

- If you are physically able but find yourself sitting in front of the computer or television for hours at a time, try to break it up and build activity into your day. You can do this by going for a short, brisk walk around the garden or in the street.

ESSENTIAL EXERCISES

Whether you're in the gym or at home, Sylvia has created a basic programme that provides balanced and ideal training for your entire body. In terms of equipment required, you can improvise with every-day household furniture such as chairs or sofa arms. If you find movement difficult, for example, then you don't have to go far to improve muscle strength and flexibility. We also find that soft drinks bottles filled with water make effective substitutes for dumbbells. Anything with a volume between 0.3 and 2 litres is effective, depending on your requirements. Finally, as a tip, it's worth winding a few elastic bands around the bottle to provide extra grip.

Essentially, what we have here are a range of dif-ferent exercises aimed at promoting strength and flexibility. You can pick and choose to suit your needs, or measure your progress by building up gradually until you can complete all the exercises in one go. Collectively, they can give your body an excellent workout, particularly if you are accustomed to doing little or no regular physical exercise. Of course, not everyone will be in a position to set out on the road to successful ageing in tiptop condition. Health issues may well play a role, but that doesn't mean exercise is out of bounds. Once again, your doctor (or the medical professional responsible for your care, should you be receiving treatment) can recommend an appropriate course of physical activity. Even if you consider yourself to be in good shape, it's always wise to get checked out before embarking on any kind of exercise as suggested here.

Squats

- Sit on a chair with your arms outstretched and feet parallel. If you're fit enough, hold a full bottle of water (0.5l or 1.5l) in your hands.

- Stand up, until your back is straight and your arms are still out in front of you.

- Sit down again.

Try to do this exercise at least 12 times without a break and increase the repetitions up to 25 times without a break.

Lunges

- Support yourself with a chair, with one foot on a cushion and your other leg stretched back, and on your tiptoes.

- Push your pelvis towards the chair, keeping your tummy tucked in and chest out, and lower your shoulders.

- Now bend your back leg towards the ground and stretch. Your upper body should stay still!

Try to do this 12 times with each leg and without a break. Increase the repetitions up to 25 times.

Push-ups

- Kneel with your hands on the floor and arms shoulder-width apart. Keep your back straight and your tummy tensed.

- Bend your arms and lower yourself until you are 10cm from the ground. Make sure your back isn't bent!

- Straighten your arms again.

Do this as repetitions of either 3×5, 3×10, 2×15 or 2×20.

Abdominal training and coordination

- Lie on your back, with both legs flexed, your feet on the floor and arms against your sides.

- Stretch one leg up into the air and, at the same time, with both hands touch your leg between knee and foot.

- Now lower your leg back to the ground and do the same with your other leg.

Repeat 5 times on each side and increase up to 25 repetitions.

Triceps presses

- Sit upright on a chair.

- Hold your water bottles in your hands and keep your arms outstretched above your head.

- Now bend your arms and lower the water bottles behind your head. Keep your elbows close together and at head height.

- Then raise them back to the starting position.

Start with an empty bottle and do this in repetitions of 10, increasing to 25. After that, increase the resistance (successively use a 0.3l, 0.5l, 1l and 2l bottle filled with water).

Stretching

- Sit with your legs out in front of you.

- Hold your arms in the air so that your shoulder and pelvis are in line with each other.

- Now try to pull your arms up into the air and stretch. Hold this position for 10 seconds.

- After 10 seconds, now try to touch your toes and hold this position for 10 seconds.

Repeat this either 3 or 5 times.

Cardio-endurance training

- Work out a route you can walk in 30 minutes.

- Walk this route quickly twice a week. To give you an idea of how quickly to walk, maintain a speed such that you can still talk with a friend – or sing if you want to! Ideally you will not be out of breath. Concentrate on your breathing; take regular breaths, breathing in through the nose and out through the mouth.

Remember to note the time you took to walk the route each time you do it.

- Work out a 60-minute route.

- Walk this route quickly twice a week. To give you an idea of how quickly to walk, maintain a speed that allows you to talk with a friend, or sing if you want to.

To make it more interesting, work in some interval training. Walk normally for 15 minutes and then very quickly for 5 minutes. Repeat this twice more. Remember to note the time you took to walk the route each time you do it.

DURING-THE-DAY EXERCISES

I like to do these exercises at home while I am watching TV or working on the computer. They don't take a huge amount of effort and they make me feel that I am not just sitting, but doing something worthwhile at the same time. Go gently with these exercises. Do not strain yourself, and stop if at any time you feel out of breath.

Ultimately, these exercises are designed for you to incorporate into your day. There's no need to set aside time. It's a question of customising any activity you do, from drinking a cup of tea at the table to standing at the hob, so it also benefits your health.

Chair march

- Sit tall.

- Hold the sides of the chair.

- Alternately lift your feet and place them down with control.

- Build to a rhythm that is comfortable for you.

Continue for 30 seconds.

Arm swings

- Sit tall away from the chair back.

- Place your feet flat on the floor below your knees.

- Bend your elbows and swing your arms from the shoulder.

- Build to a rhythm that is comfortable for you.

Continue for 30 seconds.

Shoulder circles

- Sit tall with your arms at your sides.

- Lift both shoulders up to your ears, draw them back, then press them down.

Repeat slowly 5 times.

Ankle loosener

- Sit tall away from the chair back.

- Hold the sides of the chair.

- Place the heel of one foot on the floor, then lift it and put the toes down on the same spot.

Repeat 5 times for each leg.

Spine twists

- Sit tall with your feet flat on the floor.
- Place your right hand on your left knee and your left hand behind you on the chair back or the side of the chair.
- Sit very tall, then, with control, turn your upper body and head towards your left arm.
- Repeat on the opposite side.

Repeat 5 times.

Chest stretch

- Sit tall away from the chair back.
- Reach behind you with both arms and hold the chair back.

- Press your chest forwards and upwards until you feel the stretch across your chest.

Hold for 8 seconds.

Back of thigh stretch

- Move your bottom to the front of the chair.

- Place your right foot flat on the floor, then straighten your left leg out in front with your heel on the floor.

- Place both hands on your right thigh, then sit tall.

- Lean forwards and upwards until you feel the stretch in the back of your left thigh.

Hold for 8 seconds, then repeat on your other leg.

Calf stretch

- Stand behind the chair holding the chair back.

- Step back with one leg, checking that both feet are pointing forward.

- Now press the heel of the back foot into the floor until you feel the stretch in your calf.

Hold for 8 seconds, then repeat on your other leg.

Wrist strengthener

- Fold or roll a towel (or pair of tights).

- Holding it with both hands, squeeze hard, then twist by bringing your elbows close to your body.

- Hold for a slow count of 5 – count out loud to ensure you don't hold your breath.

Repeat 8 times.

Sit to stand

- Sit tall near the front of the chair.

- Place your feet slightly behind your knees.

- Lean slightly forwards.

- Stand up, using your hands on the chair for support if needed. Progress to no hands over time.

- Step back until your legs touch the chair, then stand

tall, bend your knees and slowly lower your bottom back into the chair.

Repeat 10 times.

Upper back strengthener

For this exercise you'll need a resistance band. This is a simple fitness aid available from most high street sports shops.

- Hold the band with your palms facing up and wrists firm and straight.

- Pull your hands apart, then draw the band towards your hips. Squeeze your shoulder blades together.

- Hold for a slow count of 5 – count out loud to keep breathing. Then release.

Repeat 6 times.

Thigh strengthener

Place the resistance band under the ball of one foot.

Sit tall, lift the knee a few inches, then pull your hands towards your hips and hold.

Now straighten your knee by pushing your foot firmly downwards against the band.

Hold for a slow count of 5 (count out loud to keep breathing).

Bend the knee and release the arm.

Repeat 6 times, then change legs.

Wall press-up

- Stand at arm's length from the wall.

- Place your hands on the wall at chest height, fingers upwards.

- Keeping your back straight and tummy tight, bend your elbows, lowering your body with control towards the wall.

- Press back to the start position.

Repeat 8 times.

The following exercises will help with your balance:

Side steps

- Stand tall holding the chair.

- Take a step from side to side.

- When confident, try holding the chair with only one hand.

- Continue for 30 seconds.

Now try 2 steps to the side and back, maintaining for 30 seconds.

Heel raises

- Stand tall holding a sturdy table, chair, or even the sink!

- Raise your heels, taking your weight over the big toe and second toe.

- Hold for 1 second.

- Lower your heels to the floor with control.

Repeat 10 times.

Toe raises

- Stand tall holding a sturdy table, chair, or the sink.

- Raise your toes, taking your weight back on to your heels, and without sticking your bottom out.

- Hold for 1 second.

- Lower your toes to the floor with control.

Repeat 10 times.

Marching

- Stand to the side of the chair, holding on with one hand.

- Stand tall.

- March on the spot, swinging your free arm.

- Keep marching for 30 seconds.

- Turn slowly around, then repeat using the other arm.

Repeat 3 times.

Leg swings

- Stand tall to the side of the chair, holding on with one hand.

- Swing the leg furthest away from the chair forwards and back with control.

Perform 10 swings. Turn slowly to repeat on your other leg.

ADVANCED EXERCISES

Make no mistake, this is not rocket science. It might be a step up once you've mastered the basics, but it is in effect a series of straightforward but slightly more rigorous exercises designed to target specific muscle groups and promote core stability, and to be performed as a routine. In making your welfare a priority here, check in with your doctor first and then aim to get to grips with these exercises under the guidance of a personal trainer. Ultimately, it's about taking responsibility for your body and health, and finding a way to take care of both in a safe and constructive way.

Squats

Muscles used

Dynamic: Thigh muscles front and back, gluteus maximus

Static: All abductors and trunk

Reasons

Squats train the entire leg musculature and work the entire lower body. It is a complex exercise and requires movement in the knee and hip joints. This movement is very natural and important for older people, as it can improve your walking security.

Lunges/split squats

Muscles used

Dynamic: Thigh muscles front and back, gluteus maximus

Static: Trunk

Reasons

This exercise trains the entire leg musculature along with the hip extension muscles. It is important to keep the stabilisation of your trunk in mind, as well as the fixation of the front supporting leg. The body is not very fixed, which means that extra attention has to be paid to the correct body posture and body tension.

Training the hip extension musculature is very important for older people. These muscle groups in particular atrophy in the ageing process, predominantly through the lack of use, and so it's important to focus on this area.

Positioning your supporting leg on a cushion will also let you train your sense of balance, as well as the synergistic musculature. This exercise, too, is a complex one with movements required in the areas of knee and hip joints. As before, this movement is quite natural and important for older people, as the security and the balance of walking can be regained and improved. For security, use the backrest of a chair.

Push-ups

Muscles used

Dynamic: Pectoralis major, deltoid muscle – frontal part, triceps

Static: Trapezius muscle, abdominal musculature

Reasons

The push-up exercise is one of the most effective exercises for the pectoral musculature. As before, this is a complex exercise, and it requires movement in the shoulder and elbow joints, as well as proper stabilisation of the trunk and in particular of the abdominal musculature.

This exercise may also be performed on your knees if you are just beginning, and advanced users can perform it with stretched-out legs. Additionally your legs should be spread outwards, and only if the repetitions are done correctly should you move on to performing the exercise with closed legs.

Abdominal exercise and coordination

Muscles used

Straight abdominal muscle, outer and inner oblique abdominal muscles, transversus abdominis

Reasons

Strengthening of the trunk musculature for stabilising the trunk. A well-trained abdominal musculature relieves the spine and results in a better posture.

The training also leads to a physiological organ kneading, which improves intestinal activity.

The alternate stretching and bending of your legs, as well as the guiding of your upper body towards your leg, serves to improve coordination. The exercise can be performed with straight and opposite movements.

Triceps presses

Muscles used

Dynamic: Triceps

Static: Shoulder musculature, back extensor muscles, abdominal musculature

Reasons

Trains the triceps in an isolated fashion. Through the movement above your head, this exercise is a challenge of coordination, and the body stabilisation is higher. Strength in your arm muscles is important for older people in everyday life (getting out of a chair, getting out of bed, etc.).

Stretching

Muscles used

Glutes and lower back

Reasons

This is a very important exercise for your flexibility, as you have to perform movements along your main axis. The movement originates in the hip, requires a straightening of the back, and stretches the musculature in the back thigh muscles, as well as the back muscles.

My later life in action

In order to surprise your muscles, any training schedule you undertake must be continuously changed to be effective. Therefore, every four to five weeks my regime has to be completely redesigned. Not only does it create new challenges, it shakes up my routine and keeps me on my toes! I have my trainer, Sylvia, to thank for this. In many ways, I am a living experiment and she continues to conduct it with great results. In fact, I do not know of any other trainer who provides such rigorous standards of testing and review. All I can say is that it has worked wonders.

The table overleaf aims to provide a typical insight into the kind of training I undertake under Sylvia's watch and the performance ability it affords me. It's an excerpt from my diary, and charts nine days in a six-week programme ahead of a competition. No doubt it illustrates how carefully controlled and monitored I am by my coach, and also how little time I have for myself, which is my idea of a busy and fulfilled timetable for later life.

Day	Type of training	Content	Daily target
Monday	Fitness	Stamina training on a crossfit machine or indoor rower fitted with an ergometer (to measure energy expended during exercise). 40 minutes at a pulse rate of 110bpm Sit-ups and stomach strengthening exercises	Glutaric acidemia 1 breakdown
Tuesday	Water	60 minutes of even rowing. Pulse rate of no more than 125bpm	Glutaric acidemia 1 breakdown. Concentrate on technique
Wednesday	Outdoor	30 minutes of running or quick walking 2 × 15 minutes training with a 30-minute break between sessions	Stamina and oxygen intake
Thursday	Fitness	Strength training Balance and flexibility training	Energy, balance and agility
Friday		DAY OFF!	Recovery!
Saturday	Water	60 minutes interval training 10 mins at 100bpm, 5 mins high intensity at max 142bpm, 15 mins at 100bpm, 3 mins high intensity at max 142bpm, 10 mins at 100bpm, 2 mins high intensity at max 142bpm, 15 minutes warm down at 100bpm	Interval training
Sunday	Water	10 mins at 120bpm, 30 mins at 125bpm, 20 mins at 120bpm	Glutaric acidemia 2 breakdown
Monday	Other	Dance training	Agility and stamina
Tuesday	As previous week		

© Sylvia Gattiker

If you consider the fact that I'm doing all this in my nineties, then there's no reason at all why you can't aspire to something similar! This might seem like an intense regime, but I have been training for some time. When I first started out, I undertook a far less rigorous programme and slowly built from there.

The bottom line is that you can change your body – and it can be modified substantially. The body composition difference between a healthy twenty-year-old and a healthy eighty-year-old of the same weight is mainly that the latter has lost 50 per cent of his muscle mass to fat. By removing that fat and rebuilding muscle we can now give the eighty-year-old almost the same body composition as he had in his youth.

Health, fitness and the future

Research into some illnesses that commonly affect the aged is an industry in itself. Unfortunately, it doesn't always lead to the rate of progress we require. We still need to understand more about devastating health conditions such as Alzheimer's and other forms of dementia, and diseases such as cancer. I am still searching for an answer and doing what I can to help those who are conducting the research on their road of exploration and discovery. I avidly look at the Internet and read everything I can to try and find something new, something that will give hope to millions around the world.

In my opinion, prescribing exercise as part of a programme of preventative measures for any age-related illness or disease can only be encouraged. This isn't just on the grounds that fitness promotes and supports good health. In the space of ten years from 2001–2 to 2011–12, healthcare costs have more than doubled to £121.4 billion in the UK. The aged are probably the main cause of the enormous increase, and as we're living longer we now have compelling financial reasons to stay fit and healthy through these later years.

Unfortunately, many doctors turn to costly prescription medicines as a first line of defence, while the fitness industry does not seem ready to embrace what could be a beneficial opportunity for all involved. Certainly coaches must have the necessary training, and the exercise treatment must be covered by health insurance, but these are not insurmountable hurdles.

In some countries, doctors can sell the medication that they prescribe. Even dentists can give their patients painkillers and anti-inflammatory drugs immediately after treatment, and these are put on the bill. It is said that in some cases, medical professionals get such large discounts from pharmaceutical companies that this source can represent up to 30 per cent of their income. Could doctors in the UK be given a discount if they prescribed activity-based exercise at health clubs to their patients? It is just a thought, of course, but in facing up to this health crisis it's vital that we begin to think broadly and creatively about workable solutions.

18

The Future is Bright

We've examined the possibilities and practicalities of work, nutrition and exercise in turn. If you focus on these three components, and shape up the way you live your life, there's every chance that your future will brighten considerably. It isn't just about staying fit, healthy and occupied, of course. In many ways, successful ageing is all about your attitude to life and the opportunities it affords. So, here you'll find my general hints and tips to make sure the years ahead are happy and fulfilling.

Look after your teeth

One of the great pleasures in life is to enjoy our food, but it is crucial that we keep our teeth and gums in good condition; and, if you wear dentures, that you ensure they fit comfortably. We can keep our teeth and gums healthy by brushing them twice a day with fluoride toothpaste and by visiting the dentist regularly for a check-up. Even if you have full dentures, a regular check-up is still important because the shape of your mouth changes over time, so you are likely to need new dentures every five years.

Stop smoking

Most people know how unhealthy smoking is but, because they enjoy it, find it difficult to give up. The encouraging news is that older smokers who decide to give up have been shown to be more successful at staying away from smoking than younger people.

Even after many years of smoking, it is still worth giving up. Older people can expect a range of benefits if we stop smoking, and many of these benefits can be seen quite quickly. You are likely to be able to breathe more easily, feel better overall, find that any existing heart and lung problems are less likely to become serious, be less likely to have a stroke, recover more quickly after an operation and live longer. However, the first step is the biggest and hardest to overcome – to convince yourself that you would like to be a non-smoker.

Be good to your bones

Your genes largely influence your bone health, but it is affected by your lifestyle, too. You can strengthen your bones by doing regular weight-bearing activity (this means exercise where your legs and feet support your weight, such as walking, jogging and tennis) and by eating a healthy diet with plenty of calcium-rich foods, such as reduced-fat dairy products.

The elderly are prone to suffer a deficiency in vitamin D, which is important for strong bones. Bone tends to become weaker as we age and everyone has some degree of bone loss as they get older. Osteoporosis is the term used when bone loss makes bones significantly more fragile. It commonly affects bones in the spine, wrists and hips. It means that you are more likely to break a bone if you fall, or experience chronic pain if bones in your spine collapse.

Maintain a healthy outlook

Feeling good is not just about being physically fit and healthy. Your mental wellbeing is equally important. I also believe the two are closely linked.

In my experience, work and exercise continue to help me feel positive about myself and my place in life. We all derive pleasure from personal pursuits, hobbies and challenges, and I see no reason why we should feel compelled to give them up as we age. We might need to modify our involvement, of course, but remaining connected with such interests plays a vital role in our welfare. Without a doubt, rowing gave me the freedom to explore other avenues, and led to an interest in bodybuilding and sprinting.

Unfortunately, depression is often associated with the sense of isolation that old age can bring. While it isn't an inevitable part of getting older, pursuing an interest or exercise routine can be an important therapeutic strategy. Above all, don't hesitate to see your doctor, who can recommend an appropriate course of treatment. Your mental welfare is as important to them as your physical health, after all.

Get connected

On a basic level, if you have family and friends nearby then try to meet up with them regularly or ask them to call round. Otherwise, regular phone calls can help you to stay close. The Internet has opened up more opportunities to stay in contact, such as exchanging emails and making videophone calls. Knowing that people care about you can make a big difference to your outlook. It also provides an opportunity to get out and broaden your horizons. When you consider the rewards in terms of physical activity and mental wellbeing, it pays to make the effort.

19

Our Future is Now . . .

I hope that in reaching the end of this book you'll feel like you're facing a new beginning in your life. It could be anything from a change in perspective to a desire to reinvent yourself wholesale. If it's helped you to feel energised, empowered and inspired, then what would happen if everyone in their later years read it, took one small piece of advice and used it in their everyday life?

Ultimately, we all have a future in some shape or form. How we embrace it, and make full use of the opportunities it brings, is down to us. Should we achieve this together, then changing the way we view later life as a society is within our reach. Not only will it benefit you, but generations to come. This may seem like an ideal, but on a practical note, if your sons or daughters and their children can see the liberating effect that a drive for successful ageing can have on you then they can only respect your efforts. Frankly, the way you live your life influences others. You are a pioneer. Tread an informed, enlightened path and others will surely follow in your footsteps.

While I hope you recognise the opportunities that await us all, it's important to be aware that we have serious problems with regard to ageing that need to be addressed. The concept of retirement has resulted in huge pension liabilities that threaten our financial system. In my opinion, it's also linked to widespread chronic disease that undermines our health systems. You have the potential to rebuild both your body and your mind, and if we can make the transformation as individuals then collectively we might just make a difference for generations to come.

I am one of the few authors to write about very old age who has also experienced it for himself. I know how it feels, both as a deteriorating old soul and a rejuvenated individual with strengths I could hardly imagine I might have possessed. Since focusing on muscle building, sprinting and benefiting from a stronger immune system, I have come down with just two colds in the last seven years. In this view, I consider myself to be healthy beyond belief. In making this transformation, I've discovered that the human body is as dynamic and adaptable as the mind. We can reshape and rebuild it at any time of life, and fine tune its inner workings. We can be recycled, if you like, and lead new existences that delight us, those we love, and the world we live in. None of this is down to miracles. Rather, it's the result of hard work and a commitment to a lifestyle that promotes good health, and I've enjoyed every moment.

From here on out, I intend to continue dedicating myself to promoting the virtues of successful ageing. After all, you're the one getting old and continuing to get older. I just happen to have made that journey before you! Having arrived in good shape, I can tell you right now that the future is a marvellous place to be.

Awards

Rowing
1997–2013
40 World Masters Rowing Club Gold Medals
Life Member of Thames Rowing Club
Life Member of Leander Club

Athletics
Club: Veterans Athletic Club, London
14 Championships: 2 World Championships,
3 European Championships, 7 British Championships,
2 European Masters Games Championships
2 No. 1 World rankings

2014 (August)
Birmingham, UK:
British Champion 100m M95
British Champion 200m M95

2015
Lee Valley, London:
British Champion 60m M95, Indoors (British record)
British Champion 200m M95, Indoors (world record)

Torun, Poland:
European Champion 60m M95, Indoors (beat own British record)
European Champion 200m M95, Indoors (beat own world record)

Birmingham, UK:
British Champion 100m M95 (British record)
British Champion 200m M95 (British record)

Lyon, France:
World Champion 100m M95 (beat own British record)
World Champion 200m M95 (beat own British record)

Nice, France:
European Masters Games Champion 100m M95
European Masters Games Champion 400m M95 (world record)

Records:
4 British records, 2 world records

World record 200m M95, Indoors
World record 400m M95
British record 100m M95
British record 200m M95
British record 60m M95, Indoors
British record Long Jump M95

2015 World ranking No. 1 100m M95; 2015 World ranking No. 1 200m M95

2016
Lee Valley:
British Champion 60m M95, Indoors

Ancona, Italy:
European Champion 60m M95, Indoors (injured)

Birmingham:
British Champion Long Jump M95

Acknowledgements

I would like to express my appreciation to David Tarsh who encouraged me to attempt to write a book, to Paul Baldwin who made some sense of my ideas, and to Camilla Shestopal who, to my great amazement, found a publisher to whom I owe a debt of gratitude.

I am indebted to Matt Whyman who with extraordinary creativity has given a meaning to incidents in my life and to my thoughts on how we could change our lives.

I would like to mention Gabriela Roesch who taught me how to use a computer, without which the book could not have been written.

In addition I am deeply indebted to my coach Sylvia Gattiker who not only rebuilt my body in old age but without whom, thanks to her training and her absurd optimism, many of my athletic achievements (and my survival) would not have been possible. Sylvia Gattiker is a specialist for training in older age and you can contact her at: info@blaueshaus.ch

All those mentioned have been gracious enough to ignore my advanced old age, for which I am most grateful.

Finally I would like to express my appreciation to the Library Services of the Royal Society of Medicine, London, for their support and cooperation.

The project has enriched my life.

Charles Eugster

union hall, or the PTA. One glaring exception is so widely discussed as to require little comment here: the most fundamental form of social capital is the family, and the massive evidence of the loosening of bonds within the family (both extended and nuclear) is well known. This trend, of course, is quite consistent with—and may help to explain—our theme of social decapitalization.

A second aspect of informal social capital on which we happen to have reasonably reliable time-series data involves neighborliness. In each General Social Survey since 1974 respondents have been asked, "How often do you spend a social evening with a neighbor?" The proportion of Americans who socialize with their neighbors more than once a year has slowly but steadily declined over the last two decades, from 72 percent in 1974 to 61 percent in 1993. (On the other hand, socializing with "friends who do not live in your neighborhood" appears to be on the increase, a trend that may reflect the growth of workplace-based social connections.)

Americans are also less trusting. The proportion of Americans saying that most people can be trusted fell by more than a third between 1960, when 58 percent chose that alternative, and 1993, when only 37 percent did. The same trend is apparent in all educational groups; indeed, because social trust is also correlated with education and because educational levels have risen sharply, the overall decrease in social trust is even more apparent if we control for education.

Our discussion of trends in social connectedness and civic engagement has tacitly assumed that all the forms of social capital that we have discussed are themselves coherently correlated across individuals. This is in fact true. Members of associations are much more likely than nonmembers to participate in politics, to spend time with neighbors, to express social trust, and so on. . . .

Why Is U.S. Social Capital Eroding?

As we have seen, something has happened in America in the last two or three decades to diminish civic engagement and social connectedness. What could that "something" be? Here are several possible explanations, along with some initial evidence on each.

The Movement of Women into the Labor Force

Over these same two or three decades, many millions of American women have moved out of the home into paid employment. This is the primary, though not the sole, reason why the weekly working hours of the average American have increased significantly during these years. It seems highly plausible that this social revolution should have reduced the time and energy

Similar reductions are apparent in the numbers of volunteers for mainline civic organizations, such as the Boy Scouts (off by 26 percent since 1970) and the Red Cross (off by 61 percent since 1970). But what about the possibility that volunteers have simply switched their loyalties to other organizations? Evidence on "regular" (as opposed to occasional or "drop-by") volunteering is available from the Labor Department's Current Population Surveys of 1974 and 1989. These estimates suggest that serious volunteering declined by roughly one-sixth over these 15 years, from 24 percent of adults in 1974 to 20 percent in 1989. The multitudes of Red Cross aides and Boy Scout troop leaders now missing in action have apparently not been offset by equal numbers of new recruits elsewhere.

Fraternal organizations have also witnessed a substantial drop in membership during the 1980s and 1990s. Membership is down significantly in such groups as the Lions (off 12 percent since 1983), the Elks (off 18 percent since 1979), the Shriners (off 27 percent since 1979), the Jaycees (off 44 percent since 1979), and the Masons (down 39 percent since 1959). . . .

The most whimsical yet discomfiting bit of evidence of social disengagement in contemporary America that I have discovered is this: more Americans are bowling today than ever before, but bowling in organized leagues has plummeted in the last decade or so. Between 1980 and 1993 the total number of bowlers in America increased by 10 percent, while league bowling decreased by 40 percent. (Lest this be thought a wholly trivial example, I should note that nearly 80 million Americans went bowling at least once during 1993, *nearly a third more than voted in the 1994 congressional elections* and roughly the same number as claim to attend church regularly. Even after the 1980s' plunge in league bowling, nearly 3 percent of American adults regularly bowl in leagues.) The rise of solo bowling threatens the livelihood of bowling-lane proprietors because those who bowl as members of leagues consume three times as much beer and pizza as solo bowlers, and the money in bowling is in the beer and pizza, not the balls and shoes. The broader social significance, however, lies in the social interaction and even occasionally civic conversations over beer and pizza that solo bowlers forgo. Whether or not bowling beats balloting in the eyes of most Americans, bowling teams illustrate yet another vanishing form of social capital.

Countertrends

At this point, however, we must confront a serious counterargument. Perhaps the traditional forms of civic organization whose decay we have been tracing have been replaced by vibrant new organizations. For example, national environmental organizations (like the Sierra Club) and feminist groups (like the National Organization for Women) grew rapidly during the 1970s and 1980s and now count hundreds of thousands of dues-paying members. An even more dramatic example is the American Association of Retired Persons (AARP), which grew exponentially from 400,000 card-carrying members in 1960 to 33 million in 1993, becoming (after the Catholic Church) the largest private organization in the world. The national administrators of these organizations are among the most feared lobbyists in Washington, in large part because of their massive mailing lists of presumably loyal members.

These new mass-membership organizations are plainly of great political importance. From the point of view of social connectedness, however, they are sufficiently different from classic "secondary associations" that we need to invent a new label—perhaps "tertiary associations." For the vast majority of their members, the only act of membership consists in writing a check for dues or perhaps occasionally reading a newsletter. Few ever attend any meetings of such organizations, and most are unlikely ever (knowingly) to encounter any other member. The bond between any two members of the Sierra Club is less like the bond between any two members of a gardening club and more like the bond between any two Red Sox fans (or perhaps any two devoted Honda owners): they root for the same team and they share some of the same interests, but they are unaware of each other's existence. Their ties, in short, are to common symbols, common leaders, and perhaps common ideals, but not to one another. The theory of social capital argues that associational membership should, for example, increase social trust, but this prediction is much less straightforward with regard to membership in tertiary associations. From the point of view of social connectedness, the Environmental Defense Fund and a bowling league are just not in the same category.

If the growth of tertiary organizations represents one potential (but probably not real) counterexample to my thesis, a second countertrend is represented by the growing prominence of nonprofit organizations, especially nonprofit service agencies. This so-called third sector includes everything from Oxfam and the Metropolitan Museum of Art to the Ford Foundation and the Mayo Clinic. In other words, although most secondary associations are nonprofits, most nonprofit agencies are not secondary associations. To identify trends in the size of the nonprofit sector with trends in social connectedness would be another fundamental conceptual mistake.[4]

A third potential countertrend is much more relevant to an assessment of social capital and civic engagement. Some able researchers have argued that the last few decades have witnessed a rapid expansion in "support groups" of various sorts. Robert Wuthnow reports that fully 40 percent of all Americans claim to be "currently involved in [a] small group that meets regularly and provides support or caring for those who participate in it."[5] Many of these groups are religiously affiliated, but many others are not. For example, nearly 5 percent of Wuthnow's national sample claim to participate regularly in a "self-help" group, such as Alcoholics Anonymous, and nearly as many say they belong to book-discussion groups and hobby clubs.

The groups described by Wuthnow's respondents unquestionably represent an important form of social capital, and they need to be accounted for in any

serious reckoning of trends in social connectedness. On the other hand, they do not typically play the same role as traditional civic associations. As Wuthnow emphasizes,

> Small groups may not be fostering community as effectively as many of their proponents would like. Some small groups merely provide occasions for individuals to focus on themselves in the presence of others. The social contract binding members together asserts only the weakest of obligations. Come if you have time. Talk if you feel like it. Respect everyone's opinion. Never criticize. Leave quietly if you become dissatisfied. . . . We can imagine that [these small groups] really substitute for families, neighborhoods, and broader community attachments that may demand lifelong commitments, when, in fact, they do not.[6]

All three of these potential countertrends—tertiary organizations, nonprofit organizations, and support groups—need somehow to be weighed against the erosion of conventional civic organizations. One way of doing so is to consult the General Social Survey.

Within all educational categories, total associational membership declined significantly between 1967 and 1993. Among the college-educated, the average number of group memberships per person fell from 2.8 to 2.0 (a 26-percent decline); among high-school graduates, the number fell from 1.8 to 1.2 (32 percent); and among those with fewer than 12 years of education, the number fell from 1.4 to 1.1 (25 percent). In other words, at *all* educational (and hence social) levels of American society, and counting *all* sorts of group memberships, *the average number of associational memberships has fallen by about a fourth over the last quarter-century.* Without controls for educational levels, the trend is not nearly so clear, but the central point is this: *more Americans than ever before are in social circumstances that foster associational involvement (higher education, middle age, and so on), but nevertheless aggregate associational membership appears to be stagnant or declining.*

Broken down by type of group, the downward trend is most marked for church-related groups, for labor unions, for fraternal and veterans' organizations, and for school-service groups. Conversely, membership in professional associations has risen over these years, although less than might have been predicted, given sharply rising educational and occupational levels. Essentially the same trends are evident for both men and women in the sample. In short, the available survey evidence confirms our earlier conclusion: American social capital in the form of civic associations has significantly eroded over the last generation.

Good Neighborliness and Social Trust

I noted earlier that most readily available quantitative evidence on trends in social connectedness involves formal settings, such as the voting booth, the available for building social capital. For certain organizations, such as the PTA, the League of Women Voters, the Federation of Women's Clubs, and the Red Cross, this is almost certainly an important part of the story. The sharpest decline in women's civic participation seems to have come in the 1970s; membership in such "women's" organizations as these has been virtually halved since the late 1960s. By contrast, most of the decline in participation in men's organizations occurred about ten years later; the total decline to date has been approximately 25 percent for the typical organization. On the other hand, the survey data imply that the aggregate declines for men are virtually as great as those for women. It is logically possible, of course, that the male declines might represent the knock-on effect of women's liberation, as dishwashing crowded out the lodge, but time-budget studies suggest that most husbands of working wives have assumed only a minor part of the housework. In short, something besides the women's revolution seems to lie behind the erosion of social capital.

Mobility: The "Re-potting" Hypothesis

Numerous studies of organizational involvement have shown that residential stability and such related phenomena as homeownership are clearly associated with greater civic engagement. Mobility, like frequent re-potting of plants, tends to disrupt root systems, and it takes time for an uprooted individual to put down new roots. It seems plausible that the automobile, suburbanization, and the movement to the Sun Belt have reduced the social rootedness of the average American, but one fundamental difficulty with this hypothesis is apparent: the best evidence shows that residential stability and homeownership in America have risen modestly since 1965, and are surely higher now than during the 1950s, when civic engagement and social connectedness by our measures was definitely higher.

Other Demographic Transformations

A range of additional changes have transformed the American family since the 1960s—fewer marriages, more divorces, fewer children, lower real wages, and so on. Each of these changes might account for some of the slackening of civic engagement, since married, middle-class parents are generally more socially involved than other people. Moreover, the changes in scale that have swept over the American economy in these years—illustrated by the replacement of the corner grocery by the supermarket and now perhaps of the supermarket by electronic shopping at home, or the replacement of community-based enterprises by outposts of distant multinational firms—may perhaps have undermined the material and even physical basis for civic engagement.

The Technological Transformation of Leisure

There is reason to believe that deep-seated technological trends are radically "privatizing" or "individualizing" our use of leisure time and thus disrupting many opportunities for social-capital formation. The most obvious and probably the most powerful instrument of this revolution is television. Time-budget studies in the 1960s showed that the growth in time spent watching television dwarfed all other changes in the way Americans passed their days and nights. Television has made our communities (or, rather, what we experience as our communities) wider and shallower. In the language of economics, electronic technology enables individual tastes to be satisfied more fully, but at the cost of the positive social externalities associated with more primitive forms of entertainment. The same logic applies to the replacement of vaudeville by the movies and now of movies by the VCR. The new "virtual reality" helmets that we will soon don to be entertained in total isolation are merely the latest extension of this trend. Is technology thus driving a wedge between our individual interests and our collective interests? It is a question that seems worth exploring more systematically.

What Is to Be Done?

The last refuge of a social-scientific scoundrel is to call for more research. Nevertheless, I cannot forbear from suggesting some further lines of inquiry.

♦ . . . What types of organizations and networks most effectively embody—or generate—social capital, in the sense of mutual reciprocity, the resolution of dilemmas of collective action, and the broadening of social identities? . . .

♦ Another set of important issues involves macrosociological crosscurrents that might intersect with the trends described here. What will be the impact, for example, of electronic networks on social capital? My hunch is that meeting in an electronic forum is not the equivalent of meeting in a bowling alley—or even in a saloon—but hard empirical research is needed. What about the development of social capital in the workplace? . . .

♦ A rounded assessment of changes in American social capital over the last quarter-century needs to count the costs as well as the benefits of community engagement. We must not romanticize small-town, middle-class civic life in the America of the 1950s. In addition to the deleterious trends emphasized in this essay, recent decades have witnessed a substantial decline in intolerance and probably also in overt discrimination, and those beneficent trends may be related in complex ways to the erosion of traditional social capital. . . .

♦ Finally, and perhaps most urgently, we need to explore creatively how public policy impinges on (or might impinge on) social-capital formation. In some well-known instances, public policy has destroyed highly effective social networks and norms. American slum-clearance policy of the 1950s and 1960s, for example, renovated physical capital, but at a very high cost to existing social capital. The consolidation of country post offices and small school districts has promised administrative and financial efficiencies, but full-cost accounting for the effects of these policies on social capital might produce a more negative verdict. On the other hand, such past initiatives as the county agricultural-agent system, community colleges, and tax deductions for charitable contributions illustrate that government can encourage social-capital formation. Even a recent proposal in San Luis Obispo, California, to require that all new houses have front porches illustrates the power of government to influence where and how networks are formed.

The concept of "civil society" has played a central role in the recent global debate about the preconditions for democracy and democratization. In the newer democracies this phrase has properly focused attention on the need to foster a vibrant civic life in soils traditionally inhospitable to self-government. In the established democracies, ironically, growing numbers of citizens are questioning the effectiveness of their public institutions at the very moment when liberal democracy has swept the battlefield, both ideologically and geopolitically. In America, at least, there is reason to suspect that this democratic disarray may be linked to a broad and continuing erosion of civic engagement that began a quarter-century ago. . . . High on America's agenda should be the question of how to reverse these adverse trends in social connectedness, thus restoring civic engagement and civic trust.

Notes

1. Alexis de Tocqueville, *Democracy in America*, ed. J. P. Maier, trans. George Lawrence (Garden City, N.Y.: Anchor Books, 1969), 513–17.
2. James S. Coleman deserves primary credit for developing the "social capital" theoretical framework. See his "Social Capital in the Creation of Human Capital," *American Journal of Sociology* (Supplement) 94 (1988): S95–S120, as well as his *The Foundations of Social Theory* (Cambridge: Harvard University Press, 1990), 300–21. See also Mark Granovetter, "Economic Action and Social Structure: The Problem of Embeddedness," *American Journal of Sociology* 91 (1985): 481–510; Glenn C. Loury, "Why Should We Care About Group Inequality?" *Social Philosophy and Policy* 5 (1987): 249–71; and Robert D. Putnam, "The Prosperous Community: Social Capital and Public Life," *American Prospect* 13 (1993): 35–42. To my knowledge, the first scholar to use the term "social capital" in its current sense was Jane Jacobs, in *The Death and Life of Great American Cities* (New York: Random House, 1961), 138.
3. Data for the LWV are available over a longer time span and show an interesting pattern: a sharp slump during the Depression, a strong and sustained rise after World War II that more than tripled membership between 1945 and 1969, and then the post-1969 decline, which has already erased virtually all the postwar gains and continues still. This same historical pattern applies to those men's fraternal organizations for which comparable data are available—steady increases for the first seven decades of the century, interrupted only by the Great Depression, followed by a collapse in the 1970s and 1980s that has already wiped out most of the postwar expansion and continues apace.

4. Cf. Lester M. Salamon, "The Rise of the Nonprofit Sector," *Foreign Affairs* 73 (July–August 1994): 109–22. See also Salamon, "Partners in Public Service: The Scope and Theory of Government-Nonprofit Relations," in Walter W. Powell, ed., *The Nonprofit Sector: A Research Handbook* (New Haven: Yale University Press, 1987), 99–117. Salamon's empirical evidence does not sustain his broad claims about a global "associational revolution" comparable in significance to the rise of the nation-state several centuries ago.
5. Robert Wuthnow, *Sharing the Journey: Support Groups and America's New Quest for Community* (New York: The Free Press, 1994), 45.
6. Ibid., 3–6.

Questions for Discussion

1. What is "social capital" and how is it linked to politics? What indicators suggest that social capital is in decline in the United States?
2. What explanations for the decline in social capital does Putnam put forth? Does he offer any suggestions for reversing this undesirable trend? Does the rise in the use of the Internet bode well for the growth of social capital?

⭐ 5.4

Politics and the "DotNet" Generation

Scott Keeter

While it is to be expected that young voters would cast ballots somewhat less frequently than older citizens, who have more at stake politically at their stage in the life cycle, in most elections since 1972, when those between eighteen and twenty-one were first eligible to vote, voter turnout among the youngest part of the electorate has been in decline.

In this selection, Scott Keeter examines the participation patterns and political perspectives of the newest generation of voting-age citizens. The "DotNet" generation, so named because of their technological savvy, is a cohort of young adults

Scott Keeter is the Director of Survey Research for the Pew Center for the People & the Press.
Scott Keeter, "Backgrounder: Politics and the 'DotNet' Generation," Pew Center for the People & the Press, May 30, 2006. Reprinted by permission of Pew Research Center.

born between 1977 and 1987. DotNets formed many of their social and political impressions in the 1990s and represent a rather distinctive group for generational comparison. For example, a higher proportion of DotNets pay no attention to politics compared to previous generations of young citizens, and a very high percentage have not developed the habit of reading newspapers. But on other dimensions, the DotNet generation is less politically disengaged than the common wisdom suggests and, according to Keeter, there are signs of "a reawakening of young people to public life."

The trend in falling voter turnout among young people was reversed in 2004. The turnout of DotNets increased by 9 percent in 2004 compared to the previous presidential election. Beyond voting, this generation compares well to previous generations in terms of other civic acts such as volunteering and community activity; its members are also quite willing to express their public policy viewpoints, which lean in a liberal, pro-Democratic Party direction. In Keeter's view, "this cohort of Americans is not likely to be a silent generation."

What's the new generation coming to? Are today's young people apathetic and politically inert, as the stereotypes suggest? Are they more reluctant to get involved in politics and public life than generations past? What will American politics be like when they are eventually in charge? The answers are not what you might think. Not only is there evidence of a reawakening of young people to public life, but today's youth are politically distinctive in many ways.

First, let's be clear who we are talking about. This is not "Generation X." The youngest GenXers are turning 30 this year, and some of them are over 40 now. Instead, we are focusing on the next generation—those in their teens and 20s today—who are sometimes labeled as "Millennials," "Gen Y," or "Gen Next." . . . [We call] them the "DotNets," because of their technological savvy. Though there is no clear line dividing one generation from another, the boundary falls around 1976. Kids born after that year began coming of age in the 1990s and have experienced a very different social and political world than did Generation X, whose formative years were the 1980s.

It's true that over the past three decades, youth have been disengaging from conventional politics. In particular, electoral participation by America's youngest citizens has experienced a long, slow decline. In most elections since 18- to 20-year-olds were given the vote, voter turnout among younger Americans has fallen, and, indeed, has accounted for most of the drop in voter turnout overall in the United States during that period.

Young people have also shown other signs of disengagement from political life. In Pew Research Center polls over the past two decades, the percentage of the youngest age cohort registering a complete lack of attention to politics rose

Figure 1
Sharp Rise in Turnout of Young People in 2004

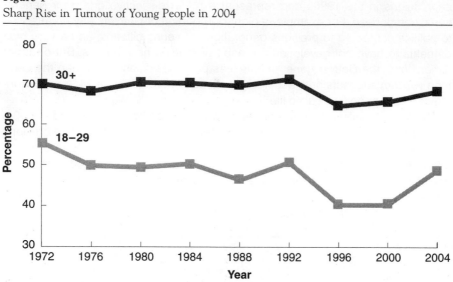

Source: U.S. Census surveys analyzed by CIRCLE.*

from 12% (in 1987–1988) to 24% in 2002–2003. Similarly, while 47% of young adults ages 18–29 were daily newspaper readers in 1972, by 2004 the number among the same age group had plummeted to 23%. Moreover, that earlier cohort has continued to read newspapers at the same rate as they have grown older (they are now mostly in their 50s). It appears that newspaper reading is a habit developed early in life. Once developed, it continues, but if it isn't started, it may never be undertaken.

The news is not all bad, however. The trend in falling voter turnout among young people was reversed in 2004. Among the voting age members of the DotNet cohort (ages 18–29), 49% voted, an increase of 9 percentage points from 2000. While young people still lag behind older adults, the rise in voter turnout among those ages 30 and older was a much more modest 3 percentage points—from 65% to 68%.

Young people were also active in other ways in the 2004 campaign, matching or exceeding the Baby Boomer cohort in several campaign activities such as displaying buttons, signs, or bumper stickers, attending rallies, or trying to persuade others how to vote.

---

*CIRCLE is the acronym for the Center for Information and Research on Civic Learning and Engagement. The center is located at the University of Maryland's School of Public Policy and is funded by grants from the Carnegie Corporation of New York and the Pew Charitable Trusts. The center's focus is on participation patterns of fifteen- to twenty-five-year-olds.